T0143817

BASIC HEALTH
PUBLICATIONS
USER'S GUIDE

TO NATURAL & SAFE PAIN RELIEF

Learn How Food and Nutritional and Herbal Supplements Can Safely Reduce Your Aches and Pains.

KENNETH J. FRANK, M.D.

JACK CHALLEM Series Editor

Series Editor: Jack Challem
Editor: Kristen Jennings
Typesetter: Gary A. Rosenberg
Series Cover Designer: Mike Stromberg

Basic Health Publications User's Guides are published by Basic Health Publications, Inc.

www.basichealthpub.com

CONTENTS

INTRODUCTION

If you have picked up this book, physical pain is probably a bothersome part of your life. Arthritis, muscular aches and pains, joint injury, back pain, and headache are extremely common complaints that could have motivated you to look for answers in this User's Guide. For some of you, pain may be disabling, preventing you from doing the things you need, enjoy, or want to do in your day-to-day life. Or, you may be looking at this book because someone close to you is in pain and you want to help. In these pages, you will find valuable information that will give you the tools and knowledge you need to reduce your pain—without shouldering the significant risks now known to exist in many of the pharmaceutical drugs normally prescribed for this purpose. You will learn how to use natural medicines—herbs, nutrients, as well as dietary changes—to reduce the impact of pain on your life.

Whatever its form, pain is the primary reason people go to the doctor. Pain Net, Inc. reports that more than 65 million Americans suffer from some form of pain at any given time, and that 90 percent of diseases are associated with pain. Pain costs the United States $100 billion a year in lost productivity, 50 million lost workdays a year, and $3 billion in lost wages a year.

Unfortunately, pain medications carry risks and side effects that range from annoying to life threatening. In 2004, with the withdrawal from the marketplace of the blockbuster pain drug Vioxx (the largest prescription drug withdrawal in history) due to sig - nificant increase in heart attack and stroke risk in patients on the drug, the public's trust in mainstream pain medicines began to wane. The safety of other similar drugs for pain has since been questioned. Although powerful corticosteroid drugs such as prednisone and sedating, addictive drugs like codeine, hydrocodone (Vicodin), and morphine are blessings for those who can't get relief any other way, they are therapies of last resort for good reason. Side effects—including addiction and major impairment of day-to-day physical and mental functioning—from these medicines can be devastating.

Now for the good news: Natural medicines—herbs, nutrients, and other supplements, dietary changes, and homeopathy—can play a role in controlling and preventing most kinds of pain. The effectiveness of these therapies varies according to the underlying diagnosis and individual response of patients, but overall they work through mechanisms that can help virtually every pain patient and that will provide complete relief for some.

With natural medicine, what helps to heal one symptom almost always is good for many other ailments. For example: Supplements and dietary recommendations that effectively treat osteoarthritis, a degenerative disease, also happen to help prevent most other degenerative diseases such as heart disease, type 2 diabetes, Alzheimer's and cancer. The same auxiliary benefits are found in natural remedies that reduce inflammation from injury. In short, all roads lead to Rome: the supplements and dietary changes I'll recommend for pain help prevent or decrease the risk of degenerative diseases as well. They fortify and strengthen the body, enhancing its natural self-healing processes.

One of the most important take-home messages of this book is that your body's level of inflammation has a lot to do with your likelihood of having to contend with chronic pain. You'll find out why this is and how stopping inflammation before it gets severe—something you can do with natural therapies—can end pain, too.

Natural approaches for pain work best when diet, supplements, exercise, lifestyle change, homeopathy, and other therapies are used cooperatively to support overall health and boost the body's ability to strike a balance that reduces pain. If you have severe pain, you may need to use some natural therapies as a complement to drugs prescribed by your medical team. If you have mild, moderate, or occasional pain, natural therapies might be all you require. *Any severe or unexplained pain should promptly be evaluated by a physician. It could signify a problem that is serious or life threatening.* Then, once you know what you're dealing with, you can use natural medicines to move toward a pain-free life.

Most of the natural pain relievers described in these pages have been used over millennia, and they rarely cause side effects—when they do, they are mild compared to those caused by drugs. Relief isn't always guaranteed with them, either, but they frequently work—without hurting you or causing addiction. They can also reduce your requirement for more toxic medicines or surgeries.

Each chapter of this book starts out with a series of simple action steps that will give you the big picture. I then go into more depth about why these steps are helpful and how they relieve pain. At each chapter's conclusion you'll find a section entitled "Dr. Frank's Natural Pain Prescription," where I sum up the advice in the chapter.

Most mainstream (allopathic) pain-care providers don't know much about natural pain relief. That is where this book comes in. It is a concise, user-friendly guide to natural therapies for pain. You can become the expert on these therapies and an important part of your own medical care.

CHAPTER 1

What's Wrong with Mainstream Treatments for Pain

All of the top ten painful diseases can be treated, at least in part, with natural medicine. Mainstream medical treatments—including the controversial COX-2 inhibitor drugs—hold significant risks. Understanding those risks will motivate you to shift to safer natural therapies.

Some types of pain respond better to natural therapies than others. Osteoarthritis, rheumatoid arthritis, fibromyalgia, athletic strains and sprains, overuse injuries (carpal tunnel and TMJ syndromes), postsurgical pain, headache, migraine, back pain, menstrual pain, and diabetic neuropathy (a potentially painful foot and lower-leg condition usually caused by diabetes) are good candidates for treatment with natural therapies. Most of these conditions are promoted or worsened by modern diets and lifestyles that don't supply adequate nutrition or physical activity.

What kinds of pain are *not* likely to be treatable with natural medicine? Pain caused by the following conditions are probably best treated with mainstream methods:

- Injury to or diseases of the nerves, brain, or spinal cord (for example, central pain syndrome [CPS], polymyositis/dermatomyositis [PM/DM], temporal arteritis, trigeminal neuralgia)

- Cancer

- Advanced arthritis or degenerative disk disease

- Endometriosis

- Internal adhesions caused by surgery

- Any pain that has gone beyond bothersome and into excruciating

There is strong evidence that intractable pain is undertreated because of fear of addiction or of being too "drugged." Don't let these fears stop you from getting the relief that will keep you comfortable.

Following is a little more detail about the top ten painful diseases treatable with natural therapies.

1. Osteoarthritis

Wear and tear on the joints leads to the deterioration of the soft, springy cartilage that cushions joint spaces. Pain and loss of joint function are the first signs of the damage of osteoarthritis. Inflammation can set in during the advanced stages of the disease, accelerating joint destruction and causing pain.

Nonsteroidal anti-inflammatory drugs (NSAIDs), such as aspirin, ibuprofen, diclofenac, and naproxen, are the first-line medical treatment for osteoarthritis. Besides the cardiovascular and gastrointestinal risks of this drug class, there is an additional concern: Research evidence shows that long-term use of these drugs actually *promotes* the progression of the disease. How ironic—the very medicine widely used to stop the pain of osteoarthritis can make arthritis worse.

2. Rheumatoid Arthritis

Like osteoarthritis, rheumatoid arthritis affects the joints. But unlike osteoarthritis, it is an autoimmune disease, an illness in which, for reasons not well understood, the immune system turns on the body and attacks body tissues and organs, including the joints.

Mainstream medical treatment usually involves NSAIDs, corticosteroids, and disease-modifying anti-rheumatic drugs (DMARDs) such as methotrexate, leflunomide (Arava), anakinra (Kineret), antimalarial drugs, gold salts, sulfasalazine, d-penicillamine, cyclo -

sporin A, cyclophosphamide and azathioprine—all with significant side effects.

The most promising therapies today are a class of drugs called TNF-alpha inhibitors: etanercept (Enbrel), infliximab (Remicade), and adalimumab (Humira). TNF-alpha is an inflammatory chemical made in the body. These drugs are given by injection, usually twice a week, and have better side-effect profiles than other DMARDs.

Natural therapies can also inhibit TNF-alpha and the enzymes that help create other inflammatory biochemicals.

3. Fibromyalgia (Fibromyalgia Musculoskeletal Syndrome, or FMS)

Chronic, widespread musculoskeletal pain; fatigue; tenderness at points along the neck, spine, shoulders, and hips; and morning stiffness (along with numerous other baffling symptoms) are characteristic of this chronic syndrome. Its causes are not known. FMS often coexists with chronic fatigue syndrome.

Pain from FMS doesn't appear to be linked to inflammation. NSAIDs have been used effectively to control FMS pain; however, natural approaches are safer.

4. Athletic/Overuse Injuries

Injuries to joints, muscles, ligaments, or bones can take a long time to mend and can turn into chronic problems. Controlling pain and inflammation naturally is a more sensible approach than using NSAIDs or stronger, addictive opiate pain medications. Supplements, dietary modifications, physical therapy, massage, and proper biomechanics, alignment, and relaxation also help athletic and overuse injuries (including carpal tunnel syndrome) heal faster.

5. Postsurgical Pain

When you return home after surgery and are ready to stop using strong pain medications, you can use natural remedies to help you get back to your healthiest, most pain-free place again.

Well before you go under the knife, be sure to talk with your medical team about which supplements you should stop using at least ten days prior to surgery. For example: some supplements (vitamin K, vitamin E, concentrated herbal anti-inflammatories, and extremely high doses of omega-3s) have blood-thinning effects that can cause bleeding problems during surgery, especially if they interact with drugs you are taking.

6. Headache

Headache can be caused by stress, muscular tension, eyestrain, sinus congestion, or dilated blood vessels along the surface of the scalp and the base of brain. Dental problems, temporomandibular joint syndrome (TMJ), side effects from medications, thyroid disease, or anemia can all cause headache. Food allergies, alcohol (especially wine, beer, and champagne), and monosodium glutamate (MSG) can too.

Some headaches require prompt medical attention. See a doctor right away if you have a sudden, severe headache, a persistent headache when you have no history of headaches, or a headache associated with any of the following:

- A blow to the head

- Confusion

- Convulsions

- Fever

- Loss of consciousness

- Pain in the eye or ear

- Stiff neck

Once you've ruled out any major issues that need to be dealt with medically, you can try natural therapies.

7. Migraine

Migraine can occur as often as several times a week or as seldom as a few times a year. Women often find that their migraines occur around their menstrual cycles, and some find that taking oral contraceptives makes their migraines worse. Intense pain may be accompanied by vomiting and may be preceded by neurological symptoms like "flashing lights."

Migraines are believed to stem from blood vessel constriction at the back of the brain, often in response to stress. As blood flow to the brain is reduced, levels of the neurotransmitter serotonin rise, causing even greater arterial constriction. To compensate, other arteries that feed the brain open wide, stimulating the release of prostaglandins that cause pain sensations. Other inflammatory responses are then triggered, increasing the pain and inflammation even more.

Migraineurs often report that stress, changes in weather, chemical fumes, flickering or glaring lights, and fatigue can bring on attacks. Others get migraines when they eat foods high in the amino acid tyramine, which is found abundantly in aged cheddar, blue cheese, most kinds of red wine, many white wines, beer, champagne, dark chocolate, and overripe bananas and avocadoes. Wheat, soft cheeses and other dairy products, yeast, food colorings, artificial sweeteners, MSG, and nitrites have all been linked to migraine. Many of these factors have also been connected to nonmigraine headaches.

In my medical practice, I told many a chronic headache patient to give up wine, champagne and beer and to develop a taste for hard liquor if they wanted to keep on drinking. This often did the trick! Other nonmedical treatments for migraine include stress reduction, biofeedback, regular exercise, and eliminating potential food triggers.

Aspirin, acetaminophen, and caffeine have helped those whose migraines are not severe. Sumatriptan (Imitrex), available as an injection, nasal spray, or pill, and ergotamine derivatives are drugs used to prevent migraine. Beta-blockers, calcium channel blockers, antidepressants, codeine or other narcotics, valproic acid (Depakote), and methysergide (Sansert) may be prescribed in cases of chronic migraine.

Acetaminophen (Tylenol) is not an anti-inflammatory; it affects the nerve impulses that transmit pain sensations. Long-term use can damage the liver, especially when used with other drugs or alcohol. And while drugs like sumatriptan (Imitrex) can be helpful, they also have harmful side effects that can feel very uncomfortable. Natural methods for preventing these headaches pose the smallest risk of side effects.

8. Back Pain

If back pain is associated with a fall or a car accident, or if you may have osteoporosis, see a doctor; you may have a fracture. If pain is accompanied by unexplained fever, chills, or weight loss, or if you have pain that grows worse when you lie down, get a medical evaluation for tumor or infection. Urinary incontinence, nerve problems in the legs, or major weakness of the leg muscles suggest nerve involvement that should be addressed by your medical team. And if back pain goes on for more than a month without resolving, it's time to get checked out.

Run-of-the-mill lower or upper back pain can respond well to specific exercises and nutrients.

9. Menstrual Pain

Research suggests that inflammatory prostaglandins are at the root of some menstrual pain. Anti-inflammatory drugs are the first-line treatment. With newly emerging questions about their safety, it makes sense to try natural therapies instead. They can work. Simple home remedies—a heating pad on the abdomen or exercise, for example—can help a lot too.

Other possible causes of pain related to menstrual cycles include endometriosis, infection, ovarian cysts, pelvic inflammatory disease, or uterine fibroids (benign tumors). These conditions do not respond well to natural therapies, and should be ruled out by a physician before trying to relieve menstrual pain naturally.

10. Diabetic Neuropathy

Not all diabetic neuropathy (diabetes-induced nerve damage in the extremities) causes pain; some people experience burning, tingling, or other sensations, and others have numbness. Since this book is about pain, we'll address the painful variety, but keep in mind that natural therapies for painful diabetic neuropathy will be helpful for other kinds of diabetic neuropathy too.

Natural medicines for this problem forestall its progression and can relieve the pain as well. Specific nutrients—in particular, alpha lipoic acid at a dose of 800 mg per day—and good control of blood sugar can help to slow down the process of nerve damage and can help rid you of your neuropathy pain.

Traditional NSAIDs: Pain Relief with a Catch

When helping a patient with one or more of these ten painful disorders, most physicians will prescribe drugs—often one in the nonsteroidal anti-inflammatory drug (NSAID) class. Although there are plenty of other drugs for pain, the majority involve high risk of an extensive range of side effects, including addiction, sedation, and liver damage. Let's look at the reasons why the NSAIDs are not the best solution for pain—and why they can, in the worst case, produce side effects that can be life threatening.

Aspirin, ibuprofen, naproxen, diclofenac, diflusinal, etodolac, flurbiprofen, indomethacin, ketoprofen, ketorolac, nabumetone, piroxicam, oxaprozin, sulindac, and tolmetin are the more popular of the traditional NSAIDs. They work by inhibiting both COX-1 and COX-2 enzymes. This inhibition decreases the production of certain types of eicosanoids—

short-acting hormones that (along with other functions) promote inflammation and pain.

The COX-1 enzyme has an important job in the gastrointestinal (GI) tract: it promotes the production of a certain type of eicosanoid that protects the GI tract's mucous lining. When suppressed by NSAIDs, COX-1 can't perform this duty, and the stomach wall tends to erode—causing gastritis (stomach inflammation) or, even worse, ulcerations that can cause life-threatening GI bleeds. I know about this firsthand, having landed in the hospital with a bleeding gastric ulcer a few years back (see Chapter Six for more on that episode).

Eicosanoids
Hormonelike chemicals that communicate information within and between cells.

Less extreme NSAID-induced erosion of the wall of the digestive tract leads to a little-known, but very common, condition called leaky gut syndrome. Corrosion of the wall of the small intestine allows substances (primarily proteins) that are not supposed to directly enter the bloodstream to do so. This can, over years, wreak havoc on the immune system, promoting food allergies and—some believe—autoimmune diseases.

COX-2 Inhibitors to the Rescue— Or So We Thought

Drug researchers reasoned that developing drugs that selectively inhibit the COX-2 enzyme, another enzyme instrumental in eicosanoid production, would prevent the estimated 16,500 yearly deaths and more than 100,000 hospitalizations attributable to gastrointestinal bleeding from long-term NSAID use. To solve this health problem, the development of the COX-2 inhibitors, including celecoxib (Celebrex), rofecoxib (Vioxx), and valdecoxib (Bextra) soon followed.

In their heyday, the COX-2 inhibitors were heralded as "super-aspirins" (despite the fact that no study had shown them to be more effective than older

NSAIDs) that eradicated the risk of GI bleeding with extended therapy (which they didn't, at least not entirely). Preliminary evidence that these drugs could help prevent colorectal cancer and Alzheimer's disease led to large, long-term studies of high-dose COX-2 inhibitors with the intention of showing them to be safe, effective preventatives.

As early as 2001, evidence began to surface that the COX-2 class might increase the risks of heart disease and stroke. By the end of 2004, this suspicion was confirmed by a large-scale study of rofecoxib. Further studies implicated valdecoxib as well. Vioxx was withdrawn from the market then allowed back with detailed warning labels about gastrointestinal and cardiovascular risks. Bextra sales have been suspended by the FDA indefinitely. So far, celecoxib—the original COX-2 inhibitor—appears to be the safest, but even old-guard NSAIDs are being reevaluated in terms of cardiovascular safety.

How does a pain drug increase risk of heart disease? When we selectively suppress COX-2 activity and the resulting production of the inflammatory, joint-destroying prostaglandin E2, the other two pro-inflammatory eicosanoid pathways remain open. These pathways, COX-1 and 5-lipoxygenase, continue to produce eicosanoids that thicken the blood and harm blood vessel linings, increasing the risks of heart attack and stroke. One theory is that because the pathway through COX-2 into pro-inflammatory prostaglandin E2 is blocked, *more* fuel goes into the other pathways—a perfect formula for increasing the risks of heart disease and stroke.

What's worse, COX-2 suppresses the formation of another eicosanoid, *prostacyclin*, also known as prostaglandin I2. Prostacyclin inhibits excess blood clotting, promotes the opening (dilation) of arteries, and helps prevent the buildup along artery walls of muscle cells that are a key element of artery plaque formation which causes heart attacks and strokes. The suppression of prostacyclin by COX-2 inhibitor drugs likely contributes to the elevated heart attack and stroke risks that have become apparent with these medicines.

Eicosanoids and their relationship to both pain and diet will be covered in depth in Chapter 2.

NSAIDs and Heart Failure

Recent research has revealed that regular use of NSAIDs (except aspirin) can double a person's chances of developing congestive heart failure, a progressive, life-threatening heart condition. A study recently published in the *Archives of Internal Medicine* suggests that the use of NSAIDs may be responsible for almost one-fifth of all hospital admissions for heart failure.

Natural Anti-Inflammatories: A Safer Approach to Pain

Preliminary results of the studies on the use of COX-2 inhibitors for cancer and Alzheimer's prevention were promising. There is strong evidence that herbal alternatives to those drugs may also have potent anticancer potential through eicosanoid control and other mechanisms that I'll describe in Chapter 5.

Questions about the safety of NSAIDs have put mainstream pain medicine in a bind. The main tool for helping people with chronic pain is the subject of doubt and scrutiny, and other medications—the corticosteroids such as prednisone and opiates like codeine, hydrocodone and morphine—have other well-established risks. Corticosteroids work by stopping all eicosanoid production, good and bad; long-term use causes osteoporosis, weight gain, radical changes in fat deposits associated with unusual body shape and facial changes, male-type body hair growth in women, immune suppression, and dependency. Opiates are addicting and mind-altering.

Now that I've established some of the risks of mainstream therapies for pain, and which disorders are best treated with natural therapies, let's move into talking about these natural therapies and how they work in the next chapter.

Dr. Frank's Natural Pain Prescription: Top Ten Painful Diseases and Mainstream Treatments

- Osteoarthritis, rheumatoid arthritis, fibromyalgia, athletic/overuse injury, postsurgical pain, headache, migraine, back pain, menstrual pain, and diabetic neuropathy are good candidates for treatment with natural therapies.

- Pain from injury to or diseases of the nerves, brain, or spinal cord; cancer; advanced arthritis; degenerative disk disease; endometriosis; internal adhesions caused by surgery; and any pain that is severe or excruciating should be treated medically—but you can still use natural medicine to complement that treatment program.

- NSAIDs, particularly COX-2 inhibitors, are mainstream medicine's main tools for treating pain, but their dangers—intestinal bleeding and raised risks of heart disease and stroke—appear to have been underestimated. Use them briefly and only if absolutely needed.

- Inhibiting inflammation with natural inhibitors of COX-2 and inflammatory eicosanoids is a major part of any pain-relief program.

CHAPTER 2

PAIN, INFLAMMATION, AND TODAY'S DIET

In this chapter, you'll find out how pain and inflammation are intimately connected and how standard American processed-food diets contribute to excess inflammation and the development of painful disorders. You will learn how to alter your diet in simple ways that will nip inflammation in the bud, decreasing your burden of pain.

When a healthy person suffers injury or infection, inflammation sets in to heal the body. This results in the attraction of many types of white blood cells and the release of immune system factors in a localized area for a brief time (usually causing pain in the process), and then dissipates, allowing healing to occur. Modern diets and stressful lifestyles unbalance the body in ways that promote excessive inflammation, either at the site of an injury or in a more diffuse fashion throughout the body. Instead of going away, inflammation can settle into the body as a chronic, slow-burning, irritating state that never quite allows healing to happen. Even minor inflammation can set the stage for more serious, ongoing pain. A small injury to the body coupled with nutritional deficiencies or imbalances can add up to a lifetime of pain.

The anti-inflammatory diet described in this chapter can be boiled down to two basic rules: eat foods that decrease inflammation (anti-inflammatory) and cut out foods that promote inflammation (pro-inflammatory).

Inflammation: The Good, the Bad, and the Ugly

Most people are under the impression that inflammation is bad, so it's important to remember that it is a natural process that occurs as the body tries to repair damage. When your body is injured or infected, inflammation sends out a clarion call to the immune system, attracting substances that battle pathogens and mop up the mess, clearing the way for healing.

Pathogens
Bacteria, viruses, fungi, or other invaders that the immune system targets and eliminates.

Inflammation can stimulate sensations of pain via both mechanical and chemical pain receptors. For example, if you have an infection beneath your skin that causes swelling, you will have pain from the pressure of that swollen area against surrounding mechanical pain receptors. Also, inflammatory chemicals released by the infection stimulate chemical pain receptors.

If inflammation occurs deep within the body, we don't see or feel proof of its occurrence. New evidence shows that a substance called C-reactive protein (CRP) is a marker of diffuse inflammation within the walls of the blood vessels—a place we don't feel inflammation. We now know that this inflammation is an important core factor in the formation of plaques that cause heart attacks and strokes.

High CRP levels are strongly linked with increased inflammation and indicate increased risk of heart attack and stroke. Autoimmune diseases like rheumatoid arthritis and lupus not only cause damage within the joints; they also involve a generalized excess of inflammation throughout the body, which causes disease in many organs. Even allergies can be viewed as a kind of chronic inflammation—an immune system reaction to a substance that is not dangerous (pollens or cat dander, for example), but that triggers red, runny eyes and nose or itchy hives.

If we understand which foods in our diet cause

Symptoms of an Inflammatory Response		
• Redness	• Heat	• Loss of
• Swelling	• Pain	function

inflammation and pain and why, we will have a better chance of making the changes that will stop our pain. But, the extent of the inflammatory response isn't *entirely* under our control. Some people's bodies are more inclined towards inflammatory overachievment. Some of us have a genetic predisposition to pain and almost all of us live in a pro-inflammatory environment (caused from pollution, disease, cigarette smoke, excessive exercise and more), neither of which can be changed. Fortunately, with diet and supplements, we can alter our bodies at the cellular level to inhibit inflammation and pain even when we've been dealt a less-than-optimal hand genetically or environmentally.

Typical processed-food diets create a tendency toward inflammation in people who would otherwise not have it and can worsen that tendency in people who are already genetically programmed to suffer from overblown or chronic inflammation. Adjusting these dietary patterns can completely get rid of pain for some people and can help control it in others, decreasing the need for traditional medications and their side effects

What is it about the foods—more specifically, the fats—in our diets that can cause inflammation to outstay its welcome. The bottom line: *Certain fats increase inflammation, while others decrease it.*

Fats in the diet directly control the body's inflammatory state by affecting the balance of *eicosanoids* (eye-KAH-suh-noyds), chemical messengers made within each of the some 60 trillion cells of the body. Eicosanoids are among the most important and potent biological substances known. These are the same eicosanoids that are affected by NSAID pain medications mentioned in Chapter One, but when, in order to stop pain, you use fats to adjust the balance in which they are produced in a more healthful direction—as opposed to NSAIDs, which block enzyme pathways so as to *stop* eicosanoid production—you do not produce the dangerous side effects associated with these drugs. The eicosanoids affect every organ system, dictating biochemical reactions in all the cells of the body, including the biochemical reactions that cause pain. They also transmit information within and between cells, affecting immune system activity, inflammation, blood pressure, blood clotting, pain, and other bodily functions.

Diet to Reduce Pain

On the grand scale of human existence, we've only had access to processed "junk" foods—a major cause of the imbalance in our diets between pro-inflammatory fats and anti-inflammatory fats—for a very brief time. We've only been sedentary since even more recently. Add to these factors plenty of psychological stress and overstimulation, and you've got a perfect recipe for pain.

Two of the drug classes widely used to treat pain—nonsteroidal anti-inflammatory drugs (NSAIDs like aspirin, ibuprofen, and naproxen) and corticosteroids (like prednisone)—work, to a great degree, by reducing inflammation. But many of the natural pain relief remedies we will recommend have broader, gentler anti-inflammatory action than drugs and do not produce dangerous side effects.

You can use diet and supplements (which you will learn about in Chapter 3) to restore a more balanced inflammatory response in your body. Eating more omega-3 fats from fish, vegetables, and flaxseeds and less pro-inflammatory fats from meat, dairy, corn/sunflower/safflower/cottonseed/peanut/soybean oils, and the hydrogenated oils are probably the most important changes you can make to help alleviate pain. Reducing your intake of all carbohydrates, especially processed sugars and flour, and consuming more antioxidant-rich vegetables and fruits will also help you reduce pain and inflammation.

A body fed wholesome food that contains all the necessary nutrients will fare better overall no matter what the cause of pain. Even when pharmaceuticals, surgeries, or other mainstream methods for combating pain become necessary, controlling inflammation with the right diet will help you along the road to recovery more effectively than if you used mainstream methods alone—or, at least, to decreased intensity of pain and a better quality of life.

Basically, if you want to use food to reduce the amount of inflammation in your body—and, by association, the amount of pain you experience—you'll need to:

- Get a proper balance of omega-3 and omega-6 essential fatty acids (all fats and oils may be referred to as fatty acids—the terms are interchangeable.

- Avoid hydrogenated oils (trans-fatty acids).

- Eat foods low on the glycemic index.

- Follow a low-carbohydrate diet (eating fewer complex carbohydrates and avoiding refined carbohydrates).

Get a Proper Balance of Omega-3 and Omega-6 Polyunsaturated Fatty Acids

There are two "families" of polyunsaturated fatty acids—the omega-3 family and the omega-6 family. Omega-6s from the food we eat are converted in the body to arachidonic acid (AA), the omega-6 fat that is then made into eicosanoids mostly of the pro-inflammatory, but also of the anti-inflammatory variety. Omega-3 fatty acids from the food we eat are converted to eicosapentaenoic acid (EPA), the omega-3 fatty acid that is made into eicosanoids of the anti-inflammatory variety only. AA and EPA are both known as "parent" fatty acids, which describes their role as the immediate precursor from which hormones are made. The eicosanoids that each parent fatty acid produces have very different effects in the body.

The eicosanoids from the omega-3 family oppose the pain-promoting actions of the eicosanoids from the omega-6 family. Therefore, the balance of these two families of polyunsaturated fats in our diets influences the amount of inflammation we experience.

The typical modern American diet contains far more omega-6 fat than omega-3. We need to eat both to be healthy, but to prevent excessive ongoing inflammation and pain, most of us need to eat more omega-3 fat (from fish, vegetables, and fruits) and less omega-6 fat (from farm-raised animals, dairy, and oils from vegetables and seeds). It is believed that the ideal ratio of omega-6 to omega-3 is between four to one and two to one, but the modern dietary ratio usually is closer to twenty to one! Our Paleolithic ancestors ate a diet with a ratio of one to one, and our genetic makeup is almost identical to theirs. Genes don't change in a couple of generations, but our eating patterns have—setting us up for a dissonance between the foods we evolved to live on and the foods we are eating from day to day.

While our Paleolithic ancestors may have had a shorter life span than modern humans, due to lack of modern medicine and the presence of saber-toothed tigers, when they did live long, they did not develop the degenerative disease we have today. Scientists have largely attributed this absence of degenerative diseases to the types of fats they ate.

Omega-6 fats are not entirely pro-inflammatory. In fact, Omega-6 fat has the potential to be anti-inflammatory in some situations unless the diet contains too many carbohydrates. Gamma-linolenic acid (GLA) is an omega-6 formed from the essential omega-6 fatty acid, linoleic acid (LA). (Essential means that our body can't make it, and we have to get it from the food we eat.) GLA is then converted to AA, which then either converts to pro-inflamma-tory eicosanoids—or, into an anti-inflammatory eicosanoid, prostaglandin E1 (PGE1). PGE1 is very good for our health. It is a powerful opener of blood vessels, inhibitor of excess blood clotting, and suppressor of viral replication. PGE1 also reduces insulin production, which helps to control type 2 diabetes, unwanted weight gain, and low blood sugar (hypoglycemia).

The amount of carbohydrate you eat determines which path GLA follows. A high-carbohydrate diet pushes the balance toward AA and the formation of pro-inflammatory eicosanoids. On the other hand, if you eat an anti-inflammatory diet that contains few carbohydrates, your body will tend to convert GLA to the anti-inflammatory eicosanoid, PGE1. Don't strive to eliminate omega-6 fats from your diet, but rather reduce consumption of those fats and raise consumption of omega-3s to improve the overall ratio in the body. Oatmeal contains high levels of GLA, but because oatmeal is a high-carb food, it's best not to rely on it entirely for your daily intake of this oil. Supplements made from borage or evening primrose oil can be a wise choice for people with excess inflammation or pain.

Fatty Acid
The most basic building block of fats and oils (liquid fats) in the diet.

An anti-inflammatory diet should also contain omega-3 fats, which be come eicosanoids that act as natural anti-inflammatories. Increasing your intake of omega-3 fats is, in my estimation, the single most helpful thing you can do to decrease painful inflammation. And doing this—in addition to eliminating trans-fatty acids from your diet—will, in time, go a long way toward decreasing inflammation and pain.

Fish is the best-known source of omega-3 fats. It contains the parent omega 3s, EPA and DHA. All vegetables, and to some degree nuts and seeds, contain omega-3s, but vegetable sources of omega-3s (including flaxseeds and flaxseed oil) differ from fish sources in some important ways. Your body has to transform alpha-linolenic acid (ALA), the short-chain essential omega-3 found in these vegetable sources, into the parent long-chain omega-3s called docosahexaenoic acid (DHA) and eicosapentanoic acid (EPA), which make anti-inflammatory eicosanoids.

It is more efficient and will do more to control your pain to get your DHA and EPA already formed as found in fish fat or fish oils than to require your body to create these parent omega 3s from vegetarian, short-chain omega-3 sources like flaxseed or its oils. Rely on fish-based omega-3s rather than vegetable-based versions if you wish to best control inflammation.

Avoid Hydrogenated Oils

Eating trans-fatty acids, found in hydrogenated oils, will create inflammation by blocking the formation of "good" eicosanoids from omega-3 fats. You'll find these fats in fried foods (like French fries), processed baked goods, chips, crackers, snack foods, and frozen dinners. Trans fats not only increase inflammation but also raise the risks of cancer and cardiovascular disease. Decrease the omega-6s, but *completely eliminate* these trans fats.

Eat Foods Low on the Glycemic Index

So far you've learned that you can improve your odds of living a pain-free life by eating a diet that is rich in EPA, DHA, and the essential omega-3 alpha-linolenic acid (ALA) and low in carbohydrates (such as bread, cereal, rice, potatoes, and pasta) and trans fats. Understanding the glycemic index (GI) will help you choose less harmful carbohydrate foods.

The glycemic index is a ranking system that tells us how quickly a carbohydrate source raises blood sugar levels, which is related to how fast it breaks down in the digestive tract and enters the bloodstream. When grains are processed into sugar (such as corn syrup) or flour, the fiber is stripped away. As a result, the carbohydrate is broken down rapidly by the body—in essence, it's predigested. On the other hand, when we eat unprocessed, whole grain, the fiber it contains slows down the rise in blood sugar levels.

Rising blood sugar prompts the pancreas to pump out insulin to escort the sugar into cells, where it is burned for energy. The higher your blood sugar, the more insulin is needed. Too rapid a rise of blood sugar often causes more insulin to be released than is needed. Excess insulin causes blood sugar levels to drop below normal levels—causing a condition of low blood sugar, also called hypoglycemia. When this occurs, you start feeling woozy, and soon you're rooting around for calorie-dense, nutrient-depleted simple carbohydrate snacks. This cycle, if repeated often, can blunt the effect of insulin and create a condition called insulin resistance: you need more insulin to move sugar into cells than you did before. A diet low in the omega-3 fatty acids EPA and DHA and high in omega-6s also promotes insulin resistance.

Insulin resistance is now understood by the traditional medical community to be at the core of weight gain, high cholesterol, high triglycerides, hypertension, heart disease, stroke, and diabetes. When some or all of these conditions occur together, doctors say you have Syndrome X (also known as metabolic syndrome). The high insulin levels associated with this condition promote inflammation and pain by disrupting eicosanoid balance.

Sugar and other refined carbohydrates rank high on the glycemic index, but they aren't the only foods that send blood sugars peaking and plummeting. Also decrease your consumption of high-glycemic fruits, grains, and vegetables, which are rapidly processed by the body. You might be surprised to find that a boiled potato has a higher GI than spaghetti; rice cakes and bananas have a very high glycemic index, although they are widely regarded as healthful foods. Fructose, or pure fruit sugar, has a lower GI than any of these foods. Get yourself a glycemic index chart—look on the Web at http://www.diabetesnet.com/diabetes_food_diet/glycemic_index.php, or purchase the book by Jennie Brand-Miller, Kaye Foster-Powell, Susanna Holt, and

Johanna Burani, *The New Glucose Revolution Guide to Glycemic Index,* available at Amazon.com and in many bookstores.

Here are some general, basic glycemic index guidelines:

- *Low-glycemic vegetables:* asparagus, broccoli, cabbage, cauliflower, celery, cucumber, green beans, leafy greens (spinach, collards, kale, chard, endive), onions, radishes, tomatoes, summer squash, zucchini.

- *Low-glycemic fruits:* apples, apricots, berries, cherries, grapefruit, oranges, peaches, pears, plums.

- *High-glycemic vegetables:* beets, carrots, corn, parsnips, pumpkin, tuber and roots (potatoes, yams, sweet potatoes), winter squash.

- *High-glycemic fruits:* banana, cantaloupe, mango, papaya, pineapple, watermelon, raisins.

Eating low on the glycemic index will do much more than reduce your cravings for simple carbohydrates like bread and sweets. It will help you drop extra weight and will protect you against developing degenerative diseases such as type 2 diabetes, heart attacks and strokes caused by artery plaque buildup, hypertension, osteoarthritis, and some cancers.

Follow a Low-Carbohydrate Diet

Eating foods that are low on the glycemic index is a great way to get started on a low-carbohydrate diet. To further reduce the amount of inflammation in your body, you should eat fewer complex carbohydrates overall and completely avoid refined carbohydrates (white flour and sugar).

Starches—complex carbohydrates found in bread and cereal—should be eaten in moderation, no more than two or three small (one slice of bread, a cup of cereal) servings per day. When you do eat bread, choose whole-grain rye, pumpernickel, pita, or sprouted-grain breads over white bread. When you eat rice, choose brown over white, and eat GLA-rich oatmeal (try steel-cut oats). When you consider that the glycemic index of many complex carbohydrates is high, you can lump a bowl of rice, potatoes, pasta or bread into the same category as a bowl of sugar. Your ability to naturally reduce your pain will hinge in large part on your willingness to decrease your intake of these as much as possible.

Some people, particularly those with symptoms of Crohn's disease or irritable bowel syndrome, should abstain from grains completely because their bodies are sensitive to them. Some autoimmune and allergic conditions can be traced back, at least in part, to a sensitivity to grains, particularly wheat. It is well worth trying to avoid grains completely for a while to see whether this improves your pain and your overall health. For some, this is the answer to controlling their pain and other health problems.

Some people with arthritis find that eliminating nightshade vegetables—tomatoes, potatoes, eggplant, squash, and peppers—helps reduce their symptoms. These people appear to have a sensitivity to these foods that affects their joints. If you have arthritis, you may wish to try this approach to reduce your pain.

Eating a low-carbohydrate diet means basing each meal around a lean source of protein: skin-less chicken or turkey, deep-water fish (anchovies, Atlantic sturgeon, bluefish, dogfish, halibut, herring, lake whitefish, mackerel, rainbow trout, sablefish, salmon, sardines, striped bass, and tuna), lamb, lean beef, tuna, legumes, or omega-3 eggs (from free-range chickens fed a diet rich in omega 3s). A three-ounce serving of meat should be about equal in size to a deck of playing cards, or one to two eggs. When enjoying fish, you can eat larger portions—up to eight ounces is fine. If you like beef, seek out grass-fed varieties, which are rich in omega-3s; grain-fed beef is much higher in omega-6 fats.

Eat Brazil nuts, butternuts, English walnuts, macadamia nuts, and others (except peanuts or cashews) as snacks. A few contain omega-3s and most others are rich in a more neutral fat, omega-9, that won't tip the balance toward inflammation.

Eat dairy sparingly, with the exception of unsweetened yogurt fermented with live cultures (preferably organic).

Use olive, or canola oils for cooking and dressings (or combine them both). They are rich in neutral fats that are not made into eicosanoids and do not produce inflammatory eicosonoids. Consider using macadamia nut oil, which is rich in omega-3s that produce anti-inflammatory eicosanoids.

Raw vegetables and fruits are packed with enzymes and anti-inflammatory nutrients that can be shut down partially or completely by cooking. You should eat some raw food every day. A big mixed-green salad once daily is a good starting point for increasing your intake of raw food. When you do cook veggies, don't overcook them; the less cooked your fruits and vegetables are, the more nutrients they have.

Dr. Frank's Natural Pain Prescription: Dietary Changes

- Build your meals around a lean source of protein: grass-fed beef and lamb, free-range organic poultry and dairy, fish, tofu, and omega-3 eggs.

- Eat deep-water, wild-caught fish at least twice a week: anchovies, Atlantic sturgeon, bluefish, dogfish, halibut, herring, lake whitefish, mackerel, rainbow trout, sablefish, salmon, sardines, striped bass, and tuna.

- Eat deep-sea fish in place of farm-raised fish; they are fed with high-omega-6 grain (usually corn), although their omega-3 content is still good.

- Enjoy as many vegetables (low glycemic) and fresh fruits (low glycemic, particularly berries) as you like; eat them raw whenever possible.

- Snack on nuts instead of refined carbohydrates.

- Use olive oil, canola oil, or macadamia nut oil for cooking.

- Take it easy on the grains (carbohydrates which include breads, cereals, pasta, and anything else made from flour), beans, and potatoes. Try not to eat carbohydrates alone in the morning on an empty stomach. This can rapidly spike your insulin levels and negatively affect your eicosanoid balance, promoting inflammation and sending blood sugar reeling, setting you up for a day of carbohydrate cravings.

- Choose whole grains such as brown rice and barley when you do eat these types of carbohydrates. Try whole-grain or sprouted-grain breads.

- Avoid grains for a while if you think you may be sensitive to them to see if your pain and overall health improves dramatically.

- Get the omega-6 oils—corn, sunflower, safflower, peanut, cottonseed, and soy oil—out of your house, along with any product that has "hydrogenated" or "partially hydrogenated" on the label.

- Try one of the high omega-3 spreads now available at grocery stores as butter substitutes.

For more details on how to implement these pain-reducing dietary changes, refer to the Resources section, which provides titles of books that will teach you how to grocery shop, cook, and eat in restaurants in ways that will decrease your pain.

If you find that you want more information about how to succeed at the approach to food, supplements, and health discussed in this book, you will also enjoy and greatly benefit from Jack Challem's book, *The Inflammation Syndrome*. This book will give you the tools you need to shop, cook, and order at restaurants so you can follow the dietary guidelines set forth here. I recommend this book to all my patients and customers with chronic pain.

CHAPTER 3

VITAMINS AND OTHER NUTRIENTS

Vitamins and other supplemental nutrients can have tremendous impact on decreasing or preventing your pain. When added to a diet that contains the proper balance of fats, nutrient supplements can reduce inflammation and pain and prevent the development of degenerative diseases. A daily high-potency multivitamin/mineral formulation will contribute to pain reduction.

Judicious and educated use of vitamin supplements (and mineral, herb, and accessory nutrient supplements) is a good idea for just about anyone. Those who stand to benefit most are the ones who have long eaten Western processed-food diets, have lived hurried yet sedentary Western lives, have diseases, take medications, and live in a polluted Western environment. This describes almost everybody I know.

Although it is unwise to take supplements instead of improving your diet—supplements can never provide you the well-rounded orchestra of nutrients found in food—the truth is that even if you eat poorly you can still experience dramatic results with supplements. Keep in mind that a good diet, an exercise program, and other lifestyle changes to reduce pain are integral parts of overall healing.

For years opponents of taking nutritional supplements claimed that you could get all the nutrition you need by eating the standard American diet. Besides the fact that nobody has clearly defined the standard American diet, another problem with this argument is that the food we eat is lacking in nutrients compared to what we ate before the development of agriculture some 5,000 to 10,000 years ago. Our food supply was further sapped of nutrients about 3,000 years ago when we began to make flour and, in modern times, by junk food and the depletion of the soil in which most commercially available vegetables and fruits are grown.

In 2001, a landmark article was published in the prestigious *Journal of the American Medical Association* (*JAMA*). It concluded that, although vitamin-deficiency diseases like scurvy and beriberi are quite rare in developed nations, suboptimal intake of certain nutrients put the general population at increased risk of developing chronic and age-related degenerative diseases.

It seems safe to assume that *optimal* is what we all want—optimal energy, optimal protection from disease, optimal repair and rebuilding of damaged tissues—not just enough nutrients to avoid vitamin-deficiency diseases like beriberi.

The average person's diet contains too little folic acid, vitamin B_6, and vitamin B_{12}, and this insufficient intake increases the risk of developing cardiovascular disease and cancers of the colon and breast. Lack of vitamin D, also common in modern diets, increases our vulnerability to osteopenia (weakened, thinning bones) and bone fractures. Failure to obtain enough antioxidant nutrients from diet is believed to increase the risk of a host of diseases, including all the degenerative diseases—many of which involve pain and inflammation.

The authors of the *JAMA* article conclude that "it appears prudent for all adults to take vitamin supplements." Although *JAMA* is one of the most widely read medical journals, the article's conclusion on supplements is one that most doctors are just beginning to recognize.

Vitamins and Supplements as Medicine: The Newest Chapter

At another level, science is finding that nutritional supplements can, in fact, be used as medicines beyond their function of filling in areas where the diet is deficient. Like medicines, supplements can produce biochemical activity in the body that can treat symptoms or cure or prevent diseases. And while pharmaceutical medicines, which are foreign to the body, do work faster than supplements in most cases, they invariably cause side effects. Supplements rarely cause such problems.

The FDA has created a set of regulations that prevents supplement manufacturers and distributors from telling you about the therapeutic medicinal value of their products. In order for a supplement manufacturer to state that a product can cure, prevent, or treat a disease, the company must apply to the federal government for that product to be approved as a medicine. This process takes an average of seven years, involves conducting numerous studies, and is likely to cost over half a billion dollars!

Drug makers go through this process routinely, and they can pay for it because their products can be patented. They can charge what they like for a new pharmaceutical agent for years after it hits the market and usually sell their products at a markup of up to 100 times or more of the manufacturing cost without fear of competition. Substances found in nature, such as supplements, are not patentable. It doesn't make financial sense for supplement makers to invest in the approval process.

Even if there is good scientific research to support a medical claim for a supplement, the FDA won't allow it to be presented by the manufacturer until the company itself goes through the approval process. For instance, the ability of glucosamine sulfate and fish oil to reduce pain in joints has been well evidenced by dozens of studies. Even so, each manufacturer of a pure glucosamine sulfate or fish oil product would have to do its own separate research and go through the application process with the FDA in order to make the claim that their product reduces joint pain!

Many nutritionally oriented scientists and attorneys believe that these limitations on health claims for nutritional supplements are more about protecting the drug industry against competition than protecting consumers against false claims. Momentum is building behind researching the medicinal value of nutritional supplements, and, as you'll continue to read in this book, strong arguments in favor of their use as treatments for painful disorders have already been established.

In this chapter, you will learn about many of the nutrients that have the greatest scientific support as pain relievers: fish oils, s-adenosylmethionine (SAMe), and methylsulfonylmethane (MSM). I'll also touch upon the importance of antioxidant nutrients, including vitamins C and E and alpha-lipoic acid, for helping prevent damage caused by inflammation. First, though, let's talk about why a high-quality, high-potency multivitamin is a good place to start, whether you are well or ill.

Multivitamins

I often tell people that they don't need a multivitamin if they eat a well-balanced diet, don't take any medications (including birth control pills), don't have any diseases, have good digestion, don't exercise vigorously, eat five servings of fruits and vegetables a day, don't live in a polluted environment, are not pregnant, nursing, or trying to get pregnant, and don't have any stress in their life. If this is you, you can skip this section. Otherwise, read on.

Many of the dosages I recommend for a basic, high-potency multivitamin are well above the Daily Value (DV) prescribed by the FDA; the DVs are guidelines for avoiding nutrient deficiency, not for supplying optimal levels for optimal health. Some dosages are well below the DV—for example, calcium and vitamin C—because it's impossible to get as much calcium, magnesium, or vitamin C as I would recommend to the average person into a multivitamin. You will have to take additional supplements for each of these nutrients—in amounts that will be covered later in this chapter.

These recommendations are based on the most-current research. Start by finding a supplement that generally matches these guidelines. A one-per-day, while better than nothing, cannot give you the optimal nutrition you will get from a multivitamin taken at three separate meals. Where there is a range for the amount of a nutrient that is recommended, according to the literature, the higher value is usually better for your overall health.

TABLE 3.1. BASIC MULTIVITAMIN GUIDELINES	
Nutrient	**Dosage per day**
Vitamin A	1,200–20,000 international units (IU)—at least 50 percent as beta-carotene and alpha-carotene; no more than a total of 5,000 milligrams (mg) of preformed vitamin A
Vitamin C	300 mg (although more is needed)
Vitamin D_3— from cholecalciferol	400 IU
Natural vitamin E— as dl-alpha-tocopheryl succinate and at least 5% mixed tocopherols (although up to 25% is ideal)	200–400 IU
Vitamin K (phytonadione)	100 micrograms (mcg)
Thiamine (B_1)	25–50 mg
Riboflavin (B_2)	20–30 mg
Niacin (B_3)	20 mg as niacin, 30–50 mg as niacinamide
Pantothenic acid (B_5)	30–90 mg
Pyridoxine (B_6)	30–70 mg
Folic acid	800 mcg

Vitamin B$_{12}$ (should equal amount of folic acid)	800 mcg
Biotin	400–800 mcg
Calcium	200–300 mg
Iodine	150 mcg
Magnesium	200–300 mg
Zinc (zinc selenomethionine)	15 mg
Selenium	200 mcg
Copper	.5 to 1.5 mg
Manganese	5 mg
Chromium	150–200 mcg
Molybdenum	100 mcg
Potassium	100 mg
Taurine	200–400 mg
Boron	2–3 mg
Choline	60–150 mg
Inositol	50 mg
Silicon	20 mg
Betaine HCl	30–50 mg

I recommend you take supplemental enzymes, which some multivitamins contain. They help break down the food you eat into its most basic components. Enzymes are produced in the body and found in fresh whole foods, but most of us don't get enough, and the result can be gastrointestinal distress and poor nutrient absorption. Some studies show that supplemental digestive enzymes help reduce pain and stiffness in people with osteoarthritis when taken on an empty stomach. Enzymes are worth checking out if other natural methods are not successful for you. One good brand is called Wobenzyme; another, by Enzymatic Therapy, is called Mega-Zyme. Take them on an empty stomach if you have osteoarthritis; otherwise, take with meals, in the dosage recommended on the container.

I also suggest you take supplemental probiotics,

a type of friendly bacteria (also found in some multi-vitamins) that live in your intestines and help break down and absorb the food you eat. Take one dose per day.

Round out your multivitamin with extra vitamin C (up to 1,000 mg per day) and 600–800 mg of calcium and magnesium.

Fish Oils

The bodies of fish that live in deep waters are rich in oils that are among the best of natural medicines for pain. These fatty acids—the omega-3 fatty acids known as eicosapentaenoic acid (EPA) and docosahexaenoic acid (DHA)—are lacking in most people's diets. I believe that this deficit is responsible for an overwhelming amount of disease, including painful diseases.

It's estimated that for controlling pain and good health the optimal ratio of omega-6 to omega-3 oils is in the range between four to one and one to one. The average Western diet's ratio is closer to twenty or more to one. In other words, we're getting far too much omega-6 and not enough omega-3. If you can achieve a one to one ratio, this appears to work best for relieving pain and inflammation; the best route to this end is taking a fish oil supplement each day.

Let's examine some of the ways that fish oil supplements can be used to treat disease. While these benefits cannot be put on the product labeling or advertisements, they have repeatedly been demonstrated in high-caliber scientific research. Remember from Chapter 2 that fish oils and the omega-3 fatty acids they contain are the best natural anti-inflammatories. Long-term evaluations of fish-based omega-3 supplements strongly suggest that adequate omega-3 nutrition, which can be obtained by using fish oil supplements and by eating deep-sea fatty fish, reduces the risk of or helps to heal a number of conditions that involve pain and inflammation. Specifically, fish oil supplements can benefit the following conditions:

- Rheumatoid arthritis (RA): RA patients have been found to have low levels of omega-3 fatty acids in their joint fluid and blood. Of all of fish oil's uses to control pain and improve tissue health, RA therapy has been the most thoroughly researched. A high dosage (at least 3,000 mg of EPA and DHA per day for twelve or more weeks) reduces pain and stiffness in RA patients and can reduce the need for medication.

- Lupus: Patients with lupus, an autoimmune disease that often involves joint inflammation and damage, may also benefit from fish oils. One small study compared very high-dose fish oil, 20 grams a day, to placebo in seventeen subjects with lupus. Fourteen showed significant improvement with the fish oils, while only four placebo subjects im proved during the thirty-four weeks of the study.

- Crohn's disease: This disorder causes autoimmune inflammation in the colon, leading to bouts of diarrhea and pain. Research using enterically coated fish oil capsules (the oils inside the capsules are not released until they pass into the small intestines, protecting the fatty acids against breakdown by stomach acids) has shown positive effects in Crohn's patients. Ulcerative colitis, also characterized by extreme inflammation in the colon, may also be helped with high-dose fish oil.

- Osteoarthritis (OA): Beneficial effects of fish oil on osteoarthritic joints were first seen in the 1950s. Those early studies used cod liver oil, which I think you should pass up in favor of fish-body oils. Cod liver oil is very rich in vitamins A and D, both of which can build up over time to toxic levels in the liver.

  DHA and EPA, when incorporated into cartilage cells, inhibit the activity of an enzyme that breaks down cartilage. More specifically, the en zyme breaks down aggrecan, a substance that confers compressibility and elasticity to the cartilage that cushions and lubricates joint movements. Other test-tube, animal, and human studies of fish oil's effects on osteoarthritis suggest that supplements could slow the disease's progression—and, as we discussed, if inflammation is involved, fish oils can help to control this factor too.

- Menstrual pain: In one study, roughly half of a group of forty-two teenaged women took a daily dose of six grams of fish oil (containing 1,080 mg EPA and 720 mg DHA) for two months. The other half of the subjects took a placebo for two months, and then the groups had their treatments switched without their knowledge. Records of their menstrual pain showed that the teens had significantly less pain while taking the fish oil. In another study, in which seventy-eight women received fish oil, seal oil, or fish oil with 7.5 micrograms of vitamin B_{12}, all groups saw improvements in menstrual symptoms, with the greatest benefits seen in the fish oil plus B_{12} group.

  Fish oils inhibit COX-2 without affecting COX-1. And remember, we learned in Chapter 2 that all three of the omega-3 fatty acids—ALA, EPA, and DHA—inhibit COX-2 production without any effect on COX-1 expression. This further supports the usefulness of fish oils as natural substitutes for COX-2 drugs.

- Osteoporosis: By improving calcium utilization, fish oils help keep bones strong.

If you are currently taking an NSAID daily or an anti-clotting (blood-thinning) drug such as Coumadin or heparin, you should not take high-dose fish oil without the guidance of your doctor. The anti-clotting affect of the fish oils added to the anti-clotting medicines may cause excessive bleeding by suppressing eicosanoids too much. Work with your doctor to wean yourself off the drugs first.

The general recommendation for good health is between 3 and 6 grams (3,000–6,000 mg), of low dose fish oil capsules per day containing a minimum of 900 mg of EPA and 360 mg of DHA. If you have chronic pain, then, at the least, double this amount. Doses as high as 20 grams of fish oil a day have been used without causing harm, although some users report upset stomach, gas, diarrhea, or a fishy after-taste with higher doses. If you are eating a portion or two of fish twice a week—one six-ounce portion is the size of a deck of cards—you don't need to take as much fish oil supplement to achieve your omega-3 goals. For each serving of fish you eat per week, you can reduce your fish oil supplements by one dose for that week.

Fish fats can be stored in the body, unlike water-soluble vitamins, which are used by the body every day. Since they are not stored, they need to be re-plenished daily. A person who isn't having pain can benefit from 7 grams of EPA plus DHA per week as a general health-preserving measure. To control pain, try for a minimum of 3 grams per day, or about 21 grams per week. You can increase this even more if needed. If you don't eat fish, to achieve about seven grams of fish oil per week, you would take:

- about three daily capsules of low-potency (about 300 mg of EPA plus DHA) capsules, which will give you about 6.3 grams of EPA plus DHA per week; or,

- one and a half daily capsules (taking one or two capsules on alternate days) of high-potency (about 600 mg of EPA plus DHA) capsules to satisfy the weekly requirement.

To achieve the three grams per day level of sup-plementation, triple the doses in the above rec-ommendations: three capsules three times a day of low-potency, or four and a half capsules (taking four or five capsules on alternate days) of high-potency fish oil.

If you eat fish, keep in mind that the fattier the fish, the better. Per 4-ounce serving, mackerel (Atlantic has 1.4 grams EPA and DHA), herring (2.3 grams), salmon (Atlantic has 2.1 grams), sardines, anchovies, striped bass, bluefish, dogfish, sablefish, Pacific halibut, rainbow trout, Atlantic sturgeon, albacore or bluefin tuna, and lake whitefish are all good sources of EPA and DHA.

For instance, if you eat a 7-ounce portion of Atlantic salmon, you get 3.7 grams of EPA plus DHA. Two of these meals a week gives you 7.4 grams. If you don't like to eat fish, supplement with enough fish oil to get your 7 grams per week. And if you want to make a bigger dent in reducing pain, increase to 14 to 21 grams of EPA plus DHA per week total between fish and fish oils. Twenty grams would be 6 fish oil capsules per day (300 mg of EPA plus DHA per capsule x 6 capsules = 1,800 mg. EPA plus DHA per day x 7 days = 12.6 grams per week) and two servings of Atlantic salmon per week (3.7 grams EPA plus DHA per serving x 2 = 7.4 grams per week).

Avoid breaded, deep-fried seafood; these foods have minimal (if any) omega-3 and are drenched in hydrogenated and omega-6 fats.

Buy fish oil that is certified free of contaminants such as heavy metals, PCBs, and pesticide residues. Pharmaceutical-grade supplements adhere to standards that ensure you are getting a pure product containing a minimum of 60 percent concentration of EPA and DHA. Most nonpharmaceutical-grade fish oils are 30 percent EPA/DHA. Fish oil supplements should contain vitamin E or some other antioxidant to prevent oxidation and rancidity. Be aware that you pay more per milligram of EPA/DHA when buying the higher concentration pharmaceutical-grade.

If you are concerned about toxicity, consider buying fish oil supplements made from anchovy and sardine body oils. These fish are lower on the marine food chain, and contain less of the toxins that tend to bioaccumulate—build up—in larger, predatory fish. You can also check with the manufacturer to confirm low levels of toxins.

One of my favorite fish oil supplements is Coromega®, an emulsified version that comes in small packets and tastes like an orange "Dreamsicle!" This product is not contaminated and studies show that its emulsified fish oils are highly bioavailable (easily absorbed into the body and into the bloodstream). Each dose of Coromega contains 350 mg of EPA and 230 mg of DHA in a highly emulsified form. Because this product has fatty acids that are highly bioavailable, this supplement provides the body the equivalent EPA and DHA of about six standard 1,000-mg fish oil capsules that each contain 180 mg of EPA and 120 mg of DHA. One packet supplies the amount I recommend daily for healthy people wanting to prevent disease and is all that is needed for most people who want to reduce chronic pain—so long as they also eat two servings of fatty fish per week. Some with greater needs may want to increase the Coromega and the fatty fish they eat by 50 to 100 percent. Those who don't eat fish and want to stop chronic pain should use at least two packets per day.

Carlson's fish oil capsules (available at www.carlsonlabs.com) are a good alternative, as are Zone creator Barry Sears's high-potency, pharmaceutical-grade OmegaRx (available at www.zoneshop.com/) and Enzymatic Therapy's Eskimo-3 (available in health food stores or online vitamin stores).

In the fall of 2005, a home test to determine your body's content of omega-6 and omega-3 will be available for under one hundred dollars. This test will determine your ratio of omega-6 to omega-3 along with other fatty-acid body-content information. You can find information about this test on www.omega3test.com.

Gamma-Linoleic Acid—The Good Omega-6

For pain and inflammation, take either 1,000–1,300 mg borage oil, 3,000 mg evening primrose oil, or 1,500 mg blackcurrant seed oil to obtain 240–300 mg of gamma-linolenic acid (GLA) per day. If you are not eating a low carbohydrate diet or if you are not tak-

TABLE 3.2. DHA AND EPA CONTENT OF COMMONLY EATEN SEAFOOD

The figures here are amounts typically found in a 3-ounce (85-gram) serving. Keep in mind that you might eat more than this—a large serving might measure 8 ounces.

Fish Species	DHA and EPA per 3-ounce serving (mg)
Anchovy (canned in oil)	1,747 mg
Crab (blue)	351 mg
Crab (Dungeness)	335 mg
Bass (freshwater)	649 mg
Bass (striped)	822 mg
Bluefish	840 mg
Carp	383 mg
Catfish	150 mg
Cod (Atlantic)	134 mg
Cod (Pacific)	235 mg
Fish sticks	182 mg
Flounder and sole	426 mg
Grouper	211 mg
Haddock	202 mg
Halibut (Atlantic and Pacific)	395 mg
Halibut (Greenland)	1,001 mg
Herring	1,712 mg
Herring (Atlantic kippered)	1,827 mg
Lingcod	224 mg
Lobster	71 mg
Mackerel (Atlantic)	1,023 mg
Mackerel (King)	341 mg
Mackerel (Pacific, Jack)	1,571 mg
Mackerel (Spanish)	1,059 mg
Mussels	665 mg
Ocean perch	318 mg
Orange roughy	1 mg
Oyster (eastern, farmed)	468 mg
Oyster (Pacific)	1,170 mg

Fish Species	DHA and EPA per 3-ounce serving (mg)
Perch	275 mg
Pike (Northern)	116 mg
Pike (Walleye)	338 mg
Pollock	461 mg
Pompano (Florida)	620 mg (estimated)
Rockfish	377 mg
Salmon (Atlantic farmed)	1,825 mg
Salmon (Atlantic wild)	1,564 mg
Salmon (Coho, canned, with bone)	999 mg
Salmon (Coho, farmed)	1,087 mg
Salmon (Coho, wild)	900 mg
Salmon (Sockeye)	1,046 mg
Sardines (Atlantic, canned in oil, with bone)	835 mg
Scallop (breaded and fried)	161 mg
Sea bass	648 mg
Sea trout	405 mg
Shrimp	268 mg
Snapper	273 mg
Sturgeon	313 mg
Swordfish	696 mg
Trout	796 mg
Trout (rainbow, farmed)	981 mg
Trout (rainbow, wild)	840 mg
Turbot	181 mg
Tuna (fresh, bluefin)	1,278 mg
Tuna (light, canned in oil)	109 mg
Tuna (light, canned in water)	230 mg
Tuna (yellowfin, fresh)	733 mg
Whitefish	1,370 mg
Whiting	440 mg

From "EPA and DHA Content of Fish Species," USDA analysis, www.health.gov/dietaryguidelines/dga2005/report/HTML.

ing enough omega-3s (specifically EPA), GLA will be converted to pro-inflammatory eicosanoids. EPA is needed for the conversion of GLA to the anti-inflammatory eicosanoids.

S-adenosylmethionine (SAMe)

SAMe, pronounced "sammy," is an accessory nutrient and a substance made in the body from the amino acid methionine. It is an important precursor for production of neurotransmitters and hormones that modulate mood and sleep quality (serotonin, dopamine, and melatonin). Since the 1950s, it has been studied as a natural therapy for depression and liver disorders. Researchers noticed early on that SAMe had an unexpected side effect: It relieved the symptoms of osteoarthritis. Based on what is known about SAMe, it has become a popular prescription drug in Europe.

The research shows that SAMe relieves osteoarthritis symptoms on a par with NSAIDs and that it causes fewer side effects. One study of forty-five OA patients lasting eighty-four days found that SAMe users got the same relief as those who took the NSAID piroxicam. Further, the piroxicam users' symptoms were more likely to return after the drug was stopped than those of the people who took SAMe.

In one study, 124 patients with migraine found that SAMe decreased the frequency, intensity, and duration of migraines. Their overall well-being improved and their use of pain medications was reduced. Studies of SAMe therapy for fibromyalgia have yielded reductions in pain, fatigue, morning stiffness, and depressive symptoms.

How does it work? SAMe increases the availability of neurotransmitters in the body that can improve mood and sense of well-being. This could explain its effects on arthritis, fibromyalgia, and migraine, or it may have some other as-yet-undisclosed positive effects that help heal joints in a more direct way and soothe pain. It is currently classified as a chondroprotective agent, along with glucosamine and chondroitin. Laboratory evidence suggests that it has anti-inflammatory and tissue-healing properties.

One catch: SAMe is expensive. It can cost $200 a month for a regular supply, and health insurers do not cover it. You stand to get your money's worth from this supplement if you suffer from depression in addition to chronic pain. Take up to 1,200 mg per day—200–400 mg two to three times daily. Don't start out with a dosage above 200 mg per day, because you might end up with gastrointestinal troubles or other side effects (dry mouth, nausea, headache, anxiety, euphoria, restlessness, and insomnia). Start low and build up to the desired dose. If you take antidepressants or have bipolar disorder, do not use SAMe.

Chondro-protective Agent
A substance that helps protect and/or rebuild joint cartilage.

Don't take this supplement at night; it can keep you awake. Take a B-complex supplement or multivitamin that includes the dosages of B_{12}, B_6, and folate recommended in the multivitamin dosages on pages 36 to 38 to prevent homocysteine accumulation that can result from SAMe supplementation. The body needs B_6 and B_{12} to make adequate SAMe on its own too, so you may find that increasing your B-vitamin intake will help your pain by boosting SAMe production.

Methysulfonylmethane (MSM)

MSM, also known as organic sulfur, is a source of the mineral sulfur that is found abundantly in the tissues, hormones, enzymes, proteins, and body fluids of humans and animals. Studies of animal models of human diseases indicate that MSM is a powerful natural pain reliever.

Soaking in sulfur hot springs is a traditional therapy for rheumatic and skin diseases in Europe and other parts of the world. Those who promote the use of MSM claim that it is useful for treatment of back pain, bursitis, carpal tunnel syndrome, headache, inflammatory bowel disorders, muscle soreness, sprains, shingles (painful blistering caused by a form of the herpes virus), strains, tendonitis, and TMJ. They say that it promotes better blood flow and has anti-inflammatory effects.

The most compelling study on this mineral thus far involved its use alongside glucosamine, an antiarthritis nutrient I will address later on (see Chapter 4). Researchers in India used a combination of 500 mg of MSM and 500 mg of glucosamine three times a day for twelve weeks in a group of osteoarthritis patients. Some subjects got only one or the other nutrient, and some got a placebo (inactive sugar pill). Scores on a standard pain index—the Lequesne index—fell from 1.7 to 0.36 (on a scale of zero as no pain and four as significant osteoarthritic pain). Glucosamine alone reduced scores from 1.74 to 0.65, and MSM alone brought scores down from 1.53 to 0.74. It's clear that the two worked better together.

Another small study, this one from UCLA, found that during six weeks' supplementation, 2.25 grams of MSM brought about improvement in 82 percent of subjects with arthritis. Only 18 percent of subjects in the placebo group had similar improvements.

The research on MSM is scant, but my patients and other doctors have reported glowing reports of its effectiveness as a pain reliever. It's inexpensive at the recommended therapeutic dose (2.25–3 grams per day), and totally non-toxic. Some people use up to 20 grams for various ailments, but this can produce bowel discomfort.

Antioxidant Nutrients for Pain and Inflammation

Oxidation is a natural offshoot of energy production at the cellular level. As your cells metabolize fuel to make energy, single electrons are split off from the electron pairs that naturally orbit the atoms that make up those cells. The loss of that electron creates an unpaired mate, known as a free radical. This is the basic process of oxidation.

Free radicals are highly reactive molecules that want nothing more than to be paired up again and balanced by another electron. They go searching for electrons to steal and may grab one from another molecule in a cell, from genetic material (DNA), from fatty acids that make up the membranes of cells, or from fats floating in the bloodstream that are bound to cholesterol. Once they get this electron, the molecule they got it from becomes a free radical, which now searches for an electron to pair up with from another molecule. This sets up a harmful chain reaction that compounds over time, causing damage to proteins, fats, and DNA, and has been linked with most chronic and degenerative disease processes.

If free-radical damage occurs in the low-density lipoprotein (LDL) molecule that carries cholesterol in our blood, the LDL becomes oxidized. This free radical damage (oxidation) makes the LDL molecule prone to deposit cholesterol in the coronary artery walls, causing coronary artery heart disease. This is much less likely to happen if the LDL is not oxidized. If free radical damage occurs in the skin tissues, it contributes to aging skin. If this damage occurs in the DNA, it promotes the formation of cancer. If it occurs in a joint, it promotes osteoarthritis.

The body has natural defenses against this electron swapping: substances called antioxidants. Antioxidants' *modus operandi* is to carry around extra electrons that can be handed over to free radicals, quenching their thirst for electrons and stopping the chain reaction causing free radical damage.

We make antioxidants within most body tissues. The liver makes large quantities of a powerful antioxidant called glutathione to help counter the high free radical production that occurs in that organ as it neutralizes toxins in the bloodstream. Good diet and a high-potency multivitamin promote glutathione production. Taking at least 500 mg of vitamin C daily can help increase glutathione production significantly. In an ideal diet, we take in plenty of antioxidant substances in the foods we eat—mostly from fresh, deeply colored vegetables and fruits.

Excessive oxidation can be caused by chronic disease, stress, hard exercise, advancing age, cigarettes, or exposure to radiation and pollutants. These elements accelerate the body's production of free radicals, increasing the need for antioxidant nutrition. So too does inflammation. In fact, inflammation and oxidation work in a vicious circle: Inflammation enhances free radical production and vice versa. It follows that preventing tissue damage and pain from inflammation requires comprehensive antioxidant protection. Not many of us eat an ideal diet with five servings of fruits and vegetables a day, and so it's sensible to supplement with extra antioxidants.

Gone are the days when nutrition experts recommended megadoses of single antioxidant nutrients such as vitamin C or vitamin E. We know today that taking an excess of one antioxidant without balancing it with others can actually increase oxidation in the body. As a result, antioxidant nutrient formulations are getting better at replicating the nutrient composition of actual foods: they often incorporate several different and complementary forms of single antioxidant nutrients.

Vitamin C, vitamin E, beta-carotene, other carotenoids, and the bioflavonoids (a class that incorporates more than one hundred different plant chemicals) are examples of antioxidant nutrients. Selenium is an antioxidant mineral that has been linked with reduced risk of chronic disease, particularly many types of cancers. Alpha-lipoic acid, coenzyme Q_{10}, and glutathione are antioxidants that are made in the body but that can also be supplemented—and there is excellent evidence that doing so is good for our health.

Carotenoids
Yellow and red pigments found in plant foods (carrots, peppers, tomatoes, leafy greens).

Alpha lipoic acid amplifies the antioxidant potential of vitamins C and E by replenishing them with an electron after they have donated one of their electrons to a free radical. Good multivitamins contain all of these except glutathione and coenzyme Q_{10}, which usually are taken separately. To promote glutathione production in the liver, I recommend increasing your intake of vitamin C. There is evidence that supplementing with too much glutathione itself can increase oxidation in people who are essentially healthy. Consult a nutritionally oriented physician before taking glutathione in quantities more than 250 mg per day.

Here are some antioxidant supplements to consider adding to your program. These dosages are in addition to those in a multivitamin. Also keep in mind that most of the herbs with anti-inflammatory activity also have antioxidant power; these herbs are discussed in detail in Chapter 5.

Some of the nutrients listed below are accessory nutrients that help the body absorb and utilize antioxidants (for example, the citrus bioflavonoids). Others also have anti-inflammatory actions that help them combat pain, and we'll revisit those later.

Dr. Frank's Natural Pain Prescription: Vitamins and Other Nutrients

- Nutrients (specifically antioxidants) relieve pain by helping control inflammation and oxidation and by helping the body's systems work optimally.

- Cover your nutritional bases with a high-potency, high-quality multivitamin.

- As part of a complete vitamin and mineral program, take extra calcium (a daily total of 1,000 mg), magnesium (a daily total of 800 mg), vitamin C (a daily total of 1,000 mg), and a B complex to meet the amounts recommended in Table 3.1.

- Supplement with omega-3 fatty acids from fish oil, which will help create the four to one ratio of omega-6 to omega-3 critical for your health and decrease inflammation. Get as much from your diet as you can (two servings of deep-sea fatty fish per week is best).

TABLE 3.3. NUTRIENTS TO USE IN ADDITION TO YOUR MULTIVITAMIN

Nutrient	Amount
Vitamin A—at least 95 percent as beta-carotene	15,000 international units (IU)
Vitamin C	600 milligrams (mg)
Vitamin E—as d-alpha-tocopheryl succinate	400–800 IU*
N-acetylcysteine (a precursor to glutathione, the powerful liver antioxidant)	250 mg
Alpha-lipoic acid ("super-antioxidant" that can donate electrons generously without becoming unstable itself)	100–200 mg
Lutein (a carotenoid)	700 micrograms (mcg)–30 mg
Lycopene (a carotenoid; tomatoes are the best source)	300 mcg–10 mg
Zeaxanthin (a flavonoid)	80 mcg–3 mg
Citrus bioflavonoids	100–200 mg
Green tea extract (contains epigallocatechin gallate, or EGCG, a very powerful antioxidant)	65 mg–2 g
Quercetin (a bioflavonoid with anti-inflammatory activity)	80–200 mg
Ginkgo leaf	60–240 mg
Grape seed extract (GSE; contains antioxidant proanthocyanidins)	100–200 mg

* Concerned about the recent studies that claim vitamin E doses above 200 IU increase risk of heart attack? Those studies didn't examine this nutrient's use with other synergistic and complementary antioxidants. If you decide to limit your intake to 200 IU or less, it should not have a large, adverse effect on your program. But plenty of evidence strongly suggests that 600–800 IU a day is strongly health promoting.

- Use a GLA supplement from blackcurrant seed oil, evening primrose, or borage oil that gives you 240–300 mg of gamma-linolenic acid (GLA) per day. Eat a low-carbohydrate diet to benefit maximally from GLA.

- Fish oils are an important part of a natural pain relief program; take enough fish oils to get from one to three grams per day of EPA plus DHA.

- Up to 1,200 mg per day of S-adenosylmethionine (SAMe) can be helpful for osteoarthritis, fibromyalgia, depression, and migraine.

- Try 2,250–3,000 mg (2.25 to 3 grams) per day of methysulfonylmethane (MSM) for any pain, particularly osteoarthritis.

- Cover your antioxidant bases by taking alpha-lipoic acid, coenzyme Q_{10}, selenium, and the others listed in Table 3.3 on page 48.

- Try 100–200 mg of grape seed extract or maritime pine bark extract especially for joint pain if your pain persists.

CHAPTER 4

GLUCOSAMINE, CHONDROITIN, AND ASU

Powerful scientific evidence suggests that your doctor's probable advice—to take nonsteroidal anti-inflammatory drugs (NSAIDs) on a regular basis—may well end up doing you more harm than good when it comes to treating osteoarthritis (OA) pain. NSAIDs may control your pain (and they don't even always do this), but ironically they make your osteoarthritis worse and accelerate cartilage degeneration by inhibiting enzymes that manufacture cartilage. The newest NSAIDs, the COX-2 inhibitors such as Vioxx, Celebrex, and Bextra may also be recommended, but these drugs have recently been revealed to pose significant dangers such as causing heart attacks and strokes, and still cause gastrointestinal bleeding associated with all NSAIDs.

In this chapter, I'll focus on the top three natural remedies for osteoarthritis: glucosamine, chondroitin, and avocado-soybean unsaponifiables (ASU). Backed by dozens of research studies, these remedies offer hope to those who would rather avoid the mainstream approach. You can use all three of these supplements together for maximum joint-protective effect.

Glucosamine, chondroitin, and ASU have been found to *promote the repair of cartilage*. No medication or surgery has ever had this effect on damaged cartilage. It might sound too good to be true, but the research evidence speaks for itself.

A recent 16 million-dollar, gold-standard, independent, multi-centered, double-blind placebo-controlled scientific study performed by the National Institutes of Health (NIH)—the Glucosamine/Chondroitin Arthritis Intervention Trial (GAIT)—has shown that glucosamine sulfate and chondroitin sulfate in combination is more effective than Celebrex in reducing pain in people with severe joint pain associated with osteoarthritis. The study also shows that individual use of each of these nutrients produces results comparable to Celebrex, but the results were better when the two nutrients were combined.

A full description of the findings was presented at the American College of Rheumatology meeting in San Diego, California, in November of 2005. The study will continue for another two years to determine whether the nutrients can reverse the tissue damage caused by osteoarthritis.

When we add this study's results to the other evidence, we have strong scientific support for their use as a natural therapy for osteoarthritis. This is breakthrough news that will, hopefully, convince skeptics in the medical and pharmaceutical community that these nutrients are tremendously beneficial and should be tried by any person who is suffering from osteoarthritis.

Glucosamine Sulfate (GS)

Glucosamine sulfate—the full name of the most-studied form of glucosamine—stops or decreases pain in joints (usually in one to three months) by repairing and rebuilding damaged cartilage. Glucosamine is a natural compound produced in the body—specifically, an amino sugar made from the amino acid glutamine and the simple sugar glucose. When linked together in long chains, glucosamine and other amino sugars create glycosaminoglycans (GAGs) and glycoproteins, which are essential building blocks of cartilage.

Cartilage
Spongy, slippery tissue that provides cushioning and lubrication within joint spaces.

Cartilage is 90 percent composed of GAGs, which in joints are in the form of chondroitin sulfates (more on chondroitin later), a type of connective tissue called collagen, and water. Supplying the building blocks of GAGs to the body seems like a logical way to help rebuild cartilage. The question remains: Does the body know what to do with glucosamine when it enters the body? When we swallow a pill full of glucosamine and it's digested, do those molecules head for the joint spaces where they're needed? The answer to this question, based on more than 300 scientific investigations that have been done on this nutrient, is *yes*.

If you want to reproduce the improvements seen in the research, be sure to take glucosamine sulfate, which is the form of the nutrient that has been researched most thoroughly. The sulfate part of the equation is sulfur, a nutrient that tends to be depleted in OA patients. Sulfur in GS helps inhibit enzymes that cause destruction of cartilage.

Two big reviews of glucosamine research were done in 2000 (at the Medical College of Virginia) and 2001 (at the University of North Carolina at Chapel Hill). Both revealed that glucosamine sulfate therapy had "moderate to large efficacy" in relieving the symptoms of osteoarthritis.

Questions of whether glucosamine is effective in long-term treatment were answered by another study, published in the British medical journal *The Lancet.* For three years, researchers followed 212 knee OA patients over fifty years of age who took 1,500 mg a day of glucosamine sulfate or a placebo. Thirty-two of the 106 patients taking placebo pills had significant joint space narrowing, compared to only 15 of the 106 GS users. This translates to half the risk of significant joint space narrowing in patients who took glucosamine. Glucosamine users had 20 to 25 percent symptom improvement, while placebo users had no symptom improvement.

How about adverse effects? Of the 106 patients on glucosamine, 21 withdrew because of nausea, diarrhea, heartburn, or stomach pain or tenderness. But 18 of 106 placebo patients also withdrew because of adverse effects—not a significant difference—and this supports that glucosamine sulfate produces minimal or no side effects. Taking the supplement with a meal is the best way to head off most side effects.

Glucosamine has no effect on blood sugar levels (although some faulty reports of research suggested this at one time) and is safe for people with allergies to sulfites or sulfa medicines (sulfites and sulfa medicines, are not the same as sulfates). People who take diuretic drugs may need higher doses of GS for the nutrient to be effective. Overall, GS is remarkably safe, even in doses well beyond the recommended 1,500 mg per day (for a person of average weight). And it's inexpensive; quality glucosamine sulfate supplements can cost less than forty cents a day.

Studies commonly compare glucosamine to NSAIDs, and overall those studies have found that patients on NSAIDs get symptom relief more quickly. Once glucosamine begins to be effective—usually in about two weeks to one month of regular use—patients on the supplement begin to show more pronounced improvement than those taking drugs and experience lower incidence of adverse effects. The positive effects of GS have been found to last for a period after patients stop taking it, unlike traditional pharmaceutical pain medications.

Glucosamine's positive effects on pain and joint movement—its two main documented effects on OA—are not achieved by blocking the activity of COX enzymes. Instead, it provides building materials for new, healthy cartilage, and it encourages the body to use those materials to fortify joint spaces. This means that it can be safely used along with NSAIDs without concerns that COX enzymes will be suppressed excessively. Of course, the goal is to completely wean off of the NSAIDs if you can.

To ease mild to moderate arthritis pain and joint stiffness, promote cartilage formation and repair, and to slow the progression of joint degeneration, take 1,500 mg per day of glucosamine sulfate. If you're an avid exerciser who doesn't suffer from OA pain, I strongly suggest you consider using GS as a preventative. Some experts suggest that glucosamine also helps promote faster healing following surgery and that it could be a helpful natural medicine for temporomandibular joint disease (TMJ) and even kidney stones. Add MSM and vitamin C to round out your program, in dosages recommended in the previous chapter.

Any person with a shellfish allergy may want to avoid glucosamine supplements, which are made primarily from crab, lobster, and shrimp shells.

Although there is not research to support glucosamine dosages greater than 1,500 mg per day (for adults), many nutritional practitioners think it wise to use an amount dependent on your weight; others say to just stick with the 1,500 mg dosage no matter what your weight.

If you don't get the results you'd like with glucosamine, and you weigh more than 200 pounds, try adjusting your dosage for your weight. Try 20 mg per kilogram, or 2.2 pounds, which is the usual amount used in the research. For example: If you weigh 250 pounds, divide 250 pounds by 2.2 to get 114 kilograms, then multiply that by 20, and you'll come up with a dose of 2,200–2,300 mg of glucosamine a day.

Chondroitin Sulfate

Chondroitin is a complex carbohydrate made naturally in the tissues of all mammals. It's a building block of healthy cartilage, just as glucosamine is a building block for chondroitin. When you take glucosamine, you're building chondroitin in your cartilage.

For years, it was said that chondroitin was useless as a natural therapy for arthritis because it was believed to be too large a molecule to absorb through the wall of the small intestine and into the bloodstream. On the other hand, several studies have shown that chondroitin is more effective than placebo at relieving pain and enhancing range of movement in arthritis patients. One study found that chondroitin subjects had more improved walking speed than subjects taking a placebo.

One meta-analysis—a type of study where data from several small studies is pooled and subjected to statistical analysis—looked at the results of four trials of chondroitin, NSAID, or placebo for osteoarthritis. Those using chondroitin did significantly better than those on placebo, particularly after the first sixty days of use. It appears that, like glucosamine, chondroitin needs some time to kick in. At the end of 2005, a $16 million National Institutes of Health (NIH) study comparing the antiarthritic effects of three treatments—Celebrex, chondroitin, and glucosamine—was presented at a national rheumatology conference. Chondroitin or glucosamine, used on their own, were each comparable to Celebrex in reduction of moderate and severe pain. When used in combination, they were better than the drug. See all the results at my website, www. DrFranksPainRelief.com.

Another meta-analysis of 702 hip or knee OA patients found that chondroitin sulfate reduced pain, improved function, and decreased subjects' need for pain medications and NSAIDs.

What is known today is that about 12 percent of chondroitin sulfate (CS) is absorbed intact through the intestinal wall. Some may be broken into smaller components in the digestive tract, allowing even more to be absorbed into the body. It is also be - lieved by many that the proper dosage ratio of GS to CS is five to four—but there isn't any actual research to substantiate this belief. The prevailing wisdom, based on the scientific research (NIH study), is that a daily dosage of CS should be from 800 to 1,200 mg no matter how much glucosamine sulfate you are taking. GS promotes cartilage formation and repair. CS appears to encourage the retention of water in cartilage and inhibits the activity of enzymes that degrade cartilage. CS may also increase production of lubricating hyaluronic acid in joints. So which should you choose?

Here's what I think: The most recent study of the NIH supports that chondroitin sulfate alone is slightly better than glucosamine alone, and that using both is best. If you can afford it, use both. Studies support that those who want the least costly route do well with glucosamine sulfate alone, especially when used with MSM and vitamin C.

Rarely reported side effects from CS include diarrhea, constipation, abnormal heart rhythms, and abdominal pain, but its overall safety profile is excellent. If you use it, take 800–1,200 mg per day.

Avocado-Soybean Unsaponifiables (ASU)

This substance has been used in France as a prescription drug (Piascledine 300 from Pharmascience) for over fifteen years to treat arthritis pain and stiffness and has documented healing effects on cartilage. And yet, in the United States, the average arthritis sufferer has never heard of ASU.

ASU is comprised of a special mixture of one-third avocado oil and two-thirds hydrolyzed soybean oil. You can't get the benefits of ASU from eating avocadoes or using soybean oil because the formula specifically uses the unsaponifiable part of the oils— that which cannot be combined with lye to form soap.

This supplement has been found to prevent the deterioration of cartilage cells that is caused by interleukins, chemicals that are involved in the inflammatory process, as well as by the damaging prostaglandin E2, one of the pro-inflammatory eicosanoids made from arachidonic acid. Test-tube studies show that ASU stimulates the synthesis of collagen, the structural matrix around which GAGs and other cartilage components are built. Other laboratory studies have found that ASU stimulates the expression of body chemicals that are associated with stimulation and repair of cartilage.

One study compared ASU plus an NSAID with placebo plus NSAID for three to six months, and the ASU/NSAID combination improved function and relieved pain significantly better than the placebo/ NSAID combination. French research showed that patients with lower-limb OA needed less NSAIDs when they also used ASU. Overall, the research on ASU suggests a persistent healing effect that lasts even after the supplement is no longer used.

ASU is available without a prescription in the United States at doses of 300 and 600 mg. No advantage of a higher dose over a lower one has been found in any of the studies. Avoid supplements labeled simply "avocado oil" and/or "soy oil." The oils must be unsaponifiable to match those used in the research. Jason Theodosakis, M.D., M.S., MPH, FACPM, a leading expert on joint health and coauthor of the bestseller *The Arthritis Cure,* offers a version called Avosoy, which can be found on the Internet and is soon to be in health food stores.

Dr. Frank's Natural Pain Prescription: Glucosamine, Chondroitin, and ASU

- Chondroitin sulfate and glucosamine sulfate used together are the best of all nutrients to heal damaged cartilage and prevent further damage. Use a dose of 800–1,200 mg per day of CS with 1,500 mg per day of GS. Since GS is cheaper, at least use it alone if spending the extra money is a problem.

- Adding MSM and vitamin C to CS, GS, either, or both is likely to enhance their effects.

- ASU is a prescription drug for osteoarthritis in Europe available in the United States without a prescription. Use 300–600 mg of ASU daily and avoid supplements simply labeled "avocado oil" and/or "soy oil."

CHAPTER 5

HERBS THAT REDUCE PAIN

Once your pain-relieving, anti-inflammatory diet and supplements are in place, you may want to experiment with some herbs that can help control your pain. If you do use these herbs, you should try them one at a time for a month or two so you can measure their effectiveness for you.

Pharmaceutical science has advanced at breakneck speed over the past century. Where once there were only a handful of drugs at doctors' disposal, there are now thousands, with a few dozen more emerging every year. Herbs—the mainstay of medical practice as recently as the early 1900s—seem all but forgotten in the race toward the next blockbuster pharmaceutical. Let's remember, however, that more than one hundred of the drugs that exist today are derived from plants. It is believed that many more await discovery, hidden away in rainforests, on mountaintops, in other natural places, and in herbs and foods traditionally used as medicines.

We are no longer sure whether medicine synthesized in a laboratory is superior to what can be gathered in nature by a knowledgeable herbalist. With modern technologies that enable us to create highly standardized, potent medicines from herbs, it appears that the sky's the limit when it comes to the potential of these drugs from nature.

Herbal medicines also have superior safety profiles in comparison with most pharmaceutical drugs. The medicinal use of herbs dates back to at least the dawn of recorded history, and the risks of using them are miniscule compared to the risks of prescription drugs. Drugs are designed to selectively influence a specific physiological activity in the body without affecting others—a sort of biochemical "magic bullet." In the real and highly complex world of the human body, however, magic bullets never quite hit their mark with exactitude. There are often unintended effects of drugs, also known as side effects.

When we try to affect only one aspect of this complex physiological world, we often end up knocking the system further out of balance. Holistic, natural medical wisdom tells us that we must treat the whole person using therapies that support the body in reestablishing a healthy, pain-free balance. Mainstream medicine tells us to eradicate disease with a magic-bullet drug or a surgery. This can work in the short-term, but in the long run it often pushes the state of imbalance that caused the disease even further.

Herbs are not highly specific magic bullets. Their actions are more general, more in tune with the way the body actually works. They are made up of many healing components often working together in a balanced way. Herbs promote balance. And this is why drugs almost always have side effects, while herbs do not.

Having said this, I want to make clear that it is possible to push beyond the balance point with medicinal herbs. (This is less likely with vitamins and minerals and won't happen with homeopathy.) They may not be as powerful as pharmaceuticals, but they are potent enough to interact adversely with pharmaceuticals. If you are at all uncertain about whether an herb is right for you, consult with an herbalist or a physician well versed in natural medicine.

Let's look again at the problems and promise of the NSAIDs currently used to treat pain. The NSAIDs range from less specific—aspirin and ibuprofen, for example—to highly specific versions like Vioxx and Bextra. (Of the COX-2 inhibitors, Celebrex is the least specific.) More specificity, when it comes to this drug class, "highly specific" means that the drug affects *fewer* of the enzymes that transform fatty acids into eicosanoids. Ironically, it is exactly this extreme specificity of Vioxx and Bextra that causes them to be dangerous.

The COX-2 inhibitors seemed to have great promise—not only for controlling pain and inflammation, but also as long-term preventatives against colon cancer and Alzheimer's disease. Until their risks became apparent, the COX-2 drugs were looking to be the next big thing in chronic disease prevention.

The most logical, safe alternatives to COX-2 drugs are anti-inflammatory herbs, which have been intensively researched and have centuries-long histories of safe use in cooking and as medicines. They can be used safely for extended periods without unbalancing the body; most of the herbs I'll talk about in this chapter *promote* the kind of balance that supports optimal health.

A great many herbs have been found to possess anti-inflammatory activity in laboratory tests. Most of those herbs have a long history of use for conditions involving inflammation. I've chosen the herbs that show promise specifically in the control of *painful* inflammation: ginger, turmeric, white willow, boswellia, feverfew, and holy basil. I have witnessed excellent results with many of these with patients who have joint pain.

Turmeric (*Curcuma longa*)

If you're only going to try one anti-inflammatory, pain-relieving herb, turmeric is the one to try. This relative of ginger has a similarly long history of safe medicinal use. It's the main ingredient of curry powder, lending it its bright yellow-orange hue, and is an important part of the pharmacopoeia of Ayurvedic medicine. Particularly, it has been used to treat inflammatory, respiratory, and biliary (related to the function of the bile system, which aids in fat digestion) disorders.

Ayurvedic Medicine
An ancient Indian school of medical thought that utilizes natural therapies to bring each individual's body into its own right state of balance.

As far back as 1971, modern medical science began to validate the traditional use of turmeric as an anti-inflammatory. The component of turmeric that has raised the most interest is a compound called curcumin. Curcumin is an anti-inflammatory that has been described by some as 50 percent as strong as cortisone, which is one of modern medicine's most potent anti-inflammatory agents. Cortisone is used sparingly because it can cause some dangerous side effects, none of which have been associated with curcumin.

Laboratory studies have identified several inflammatory pathways that are inhibited by curcumin, including two of the pro-inflammatory eicosanoid pathways and other inflammatory biochemicals—called *cytokines*—such as tumor necrosis factor (TNF) and interleukin-12 (IL-12).

Here are some other points to consider about turmeric and curcumin:

- Turmeric (curcumin) has long been used as a food preservative. It is a powerful antioxidant, even more so than the most popular form of vitamin E. Feeding turmeric to lab animals lowers their body levels of free radicals significantly.

- Curcumin is being aggressively investigated as an anticarcinogen.

- In an experimental model of inflammatory bowel disease (IBD), inflammatory markers were significantly decreased in the colons of mice with IBD who received curcumin supplementation. Other research shows that curcumin also helps relieve intestinal inflammation caused by colitis.

- Curcumin has blood-sugar lowering effects, which are beneficial for people with diabetes or pre - diabetes.

- In one study, a group of patients were given either 400 mg of curcumin, placebo, or an anti-inflamma - tory drug (phenylbutazone) three times a day for five days following surgery or trauma. Curcumin was as effective as phenylbutazone (a powerful pain reliever with strong side effects) in reducing postsurgical inflammation.

- When forty-nine rheumatoid arthritis patients were given 1,200 mg per day of curcumin for five to six weeks, their morning stiffness was reduced and their physical endurance was enhanced.

If you are generally healthy, adding turmeric to foods—using curry powder in sauces and marinades is a good way to do this—will help you stay that way. Or, try taking turmeric powder in capsules. Turmeric powder does not contain enough curcumin to match the amounts successfully used to relieve inflammation. Consider taking a supplement in doses of 100–300 mg of powdered extract standardized to 95 percent curcumin three times a day with meals, or a standardized liquid extract in gelatin capsules. I recommend a curcumin product called Curcumin C3 Complex, made by Sabinsa—a company that adheres to the highest standards. Curcumin C3 Complex is available in health food stores and through many online retailers.

Ginger (*Zingiber officinale*)

Ancient Greeks and Romans used ginger as a spice; according to tax records from Rome in the second century A.D., ginger was an important source of income for the Roman treasury. Chinese medical texts dating back to the fourth century B.C. describe this pungent herb's use in treatment of arthritis, stomachache, nausea, toothache, and bleeding problems. Ginger is used today by herbalists to treat coughs and other respiratory conditions, and it has an excellent track record as a treatment for motion sickness and postsurgical and pregnancy-related nausea. It's an effective folk remedy for the cramping of colic and intestinal gas.

Since the COX-2 drug recalls, the body of research on this herb's anti-inflammatory potential has come to light. Ginger inhibits both COX enzymes and the 5-lipoxygenase enzyme. This means that it has a broader spectrum of anti-inflammatory and pain-relieving activity compared to most NSAIDs, which don't inhibit all of these pathways at the same time. It also inhibits platelet aggregation, the clumping together of blood platelets that is enhanced by drugs like Vioxx. Some findings from the research about the potential of this natural anti-inflammatory are summarized here.

- Ginger supplements inhibited paw swelling in an animal model of arthritis, working as well as aspirin in this regard.

- Some research indicates that ginger is an effective reliever of pain related to menstrual periods.

- One study found that 75 percent of patients with osteoarthritis and rheumatoid arthritis got relief from pain and swelling in the joints with daily dried-ginger supplementation. All involved patients who had muscular pain found that pain relieved when they used ginger.

- Extensive laboratory research shows that phytochemicals in ginger have significant antioxidant capacity.

- One preliminary study reported that 74 percent of the twenty-eight patients with rheumatoid arthritis reported marked improvement in pain after taking 1–2 grams of powdered ginger per day for up to two and half years.

- Fresh ginger is rich in an enzyme called protease, which has anti-inflammatory activity.

- Laboratory studies have shown that ginger chemicals inhibit the release of substance P, a biochemical that stimulates pain sensations in the body.

- Ginger has antiulcer properties. It can protect against ulcers caused by the NSAID indomethacin, aspirin, and alcohol.

- Other research suggests that ginger may help prevent or relieve migraine headaches.

Start by buying some fresh ginger at the market and cooking with it. Asian cuisine uses lots of ginger. Try ginger tea made from store-bought tea bags or sliced or grated ginger root that you boil, steep (for 5–10 minutes), and strain into your teacup. To use ginger as a medicine for pain from arthritis, menstrual periods, or migraine, take one-half to three-quarters of a teaspoon of powdered ginger up to three times a day; or, take a one-quarter to one-half inch thick slice of fresh ginger up to three times daily. Crystallized ginger, which is sweet, can also be used; chew two pieces a day.

If you don't like the taste of ginger, seek out a ginger extract supplement that is standardized to contain high doses of the herb's active constituents. Try 100–200 mg every four hours or three times daily. For sore muscles or joints you can massage the area with a combination of ginger oil and a neutral oil such as sweet almond or light olive oil.

Pregnant women are cautioned against using more than 2 grams of ginger a day. If you take blood-thinning medications or are taking an NSAID regularly, check with your doctor before using ginger in higher doses than you would use as a seasoning.

Boswellia (*Boswellia serrata*)

This herb is a close relative of the frankincense toted through the desert by the wisemen, and it has been an important Ayurvedic medicine for hundreds of years. The gum of the Boswellia tree, called *guggulu*, contains active constituents known collectively as boswellic acids. Standardized preparations made from *guggulu* have been researched for the treatment of osteoarthritis, rheumatoid arthritis, ulcerative colitis, Crohn's disease, and asthma.

Overall, this herb appears to hold enormous promise as a natural anti-inflammatory. Test-tube studies have shown that it is a powerful inhibitor of 5-lipoxygenase (5-LO) activity, blocking the formation of the pro-inflammatory eicosanoids leukotriene B4 and 5-HETE. Both of these substances are known to play a role in the swelling and increased blood flow that characterize inflammation—and, interestingly, in the airway swelling characteristic of asthma.

A few pieces of promising boswellia research:

- Patients with ulcerative colitis were given either boswellia extract or the powerful drug sulfasalazine. Both groups showed similar improvements.

- Crohn's disease patients took either boswellia or the drug mesalazine to treat their symptoms; both groups had comparable improvements.

- Animal models of arthritis have shown that boswellic acids work to relieve joint inflammation by inhibiting the production of inflammatory mediators, blocking mechanisms that reduce production of glycosaminoglycans (GAGs) and improving circulation within joint tissues.

- A combination of curcumin and *Boswellia serrata* (a total of 500 mg taken every eight hours for three months) was tested as a therapy for knee osteoarthritis. This herbal one-two punch proved quite effective at reducing pain caused by both active and passive movements. Fluid accumulation was reduced in the affected joint, as were markers of inflammation and oxidation. Levels of powerful antioxidant substances rose in the bloodstream. The placebo group in this study showed no measurable improvement.

- Another study of knee OA showed improvement with boswellia alone, reporting decreased swelling and pain and improved function. Patients saw symptoms return when the placebo and boswellia groups were switched (those who had been using boswellia were put on placebo and vice versa).

Choose a standardized extract that contains 37.5 to 65 percent boswellic acids. Take 200–400 mg three times daily; you can use up to 1,200 mg three times a day safely. It may take a month or more to start feeling a difference. Rarely, side effects—stomach pain, diarrhea, and rash—have been reported.

Feverfew (*Tanacetum parthenium*)

Although its name is adapted from the Latin for "fever reducer," feverfew has become the alternative remedy of choice for an affliction that does not involve fever at all: migraine.

Feverfew is a member of the sunflower family, and it has been used traditionally to treat asthma, difficult labors, irregular menstruation, and skin conditions. In the 1980s, a study of British migraine sufferers revealed that eating fresh feverfew leaves daily created substantial improvement in 70 percent of the subjects.

More recently, a review article on feverfew for migraine prevention found that three of five studies showed significant reductions in migraine frequency, pain intensity, and the incidence and severity of nausea and vomiting. Two other trials showed no effect within two to four months of daily feverfew.

Overall, the research evidence in favor of this herb as a migraine preventative isn't conclusive. (Neither is the evidence in favor of many of the drugs commonly used to prevent migraines.) Its risks are minimal compared to those of migraine drugs, so it may be worthwhile to give feverfew a try if your current program isn't keeping up with your headaches.

The active constituent of feverfew is believed to be a plant chemical called parthenolide, which inhibits blood-vessel constriction, serotonin activity, and blood clotting—all elements that combine to create migraines. Among feverfew preparations, which are available as teas, capsules, tinctures, tablets, and liquids, the amount of parthenolide can vary dramatically. Look for a preparation that is standardized to 0.2 percent parthenolide. Take 100–250 mg one to three times per day, or eat one to three fresh leaves one to three times a day. Be patient—the herb can take a month or more to be-come effective.

Feverfew can interact with antiplatelet and antico-agulant medications. Don't use it if you are pregnant or nursing.

Holy Basil (*Ocimum sanctum*)

Ayurveda holds holy basil—which in Sanskrit is known as *tulsi*—in high esteem, classifying it among the most powerful of the medicinal plants. It is said to promote perfect health, long life, and enlighten-ment. Modern nutritional analysis of this variety of basil, which is not traditionally used in cooking, lends support to Ayurveda's high regard.

Holy basil contains several active constituents with documented antioxidant, anti-inflammatory activity, including eugenol, ursolic acid, rosmarinic acid (also found in rosemary, another herb believed to have anti-inflammatory properties), and apigenin. Test-tube experiments show that ursolic acid is a powerful inhibitor of the COX-2 enzyme and that it could help to prevent cancer as well as relieve pain and inflammation.

Animal research shows that holy basil relieves pain as well as a standard dose of aspirin and other NSAIDs, including naproxen—not surprising in light of *tulsi's* long history of use for treating arthritis in Ayurvedic medicine. Animal research shows that holy basil phytochemicals reduce inflammation caused by arachidonic acid and leukotrienes. Test-tube studies of breast cancer cells show significant anti-COX-2 activity of holy basil phytochemicals.

Holy basil is also effective at reducing the impact of stress on the body; it is an adaptogen that increas-es stamina and enhances immune activity. A study published in the *Indian Journal of Pharmacology* found that holy basil was a more effective adaptogen than Siberian ginseng or *Panax* ginseng, two popu-lar adaptogenic herbs that have been intensively researched. Adaptogenic effects are helpful to those who struggle with the stressful problem of chronic pain.

People in pain will almost universally benefit from

holy basil. It targets inflammation in many ways. Avoid it during pregnancy and lactation, and don't use it if you are trying to get pregnant (early studies suggested a mild antifertility effect). Do not give medicinal doses of holy basil to infants or toddlers. People with diabetes may benefit from holy basil's hypoglycemic (blood-sugar lowering) effects, but these same effects may cause problems in people who tend to have low blood-sugar "crashes" or diabetics on blood-sugar lowering drugs or insulin. Check with your doctor if you have any of these concerns.

Traditional use of *tulsi* is as a tea. You can also try 1–2 grams per day of dried-leaf capsules. Allow a week to a month for the herb's effects to kick in.

Summing Up: Herbs for Pain and Inflammation

There are too many herbs with anti-inflammatory and antioxidant activity to discuss them all in this short chapter. I've discussed the ones supported by the most evidence, but others are worth considering: green tea, Baikal scullcap, hu zhang (a Chinese medicinal herb), German chamomile, licorice, echinacea, rosemary, stinging nettle, devil's claw, and cayenne all have documented anti-inflammatory properties. If you wish to investigate further the potential for treating your pain with herbs, consult with an herbalist, or with a nutritionally oriented or naturopathic physician; or, browse the section on herbal medicine in your bookstore or health food store.

Dr. Frank's Natural Pain Prescription: Herbs That Reduce Pain

- Herbs with anti-inflammatory action are safe alternatives to NSAIDs.

- You can use some or all of the herbs in this chapter. Use them in cooking or take them as supplements or teas. Combination formulas are available in health food stores.

- Try one herb for one to two months to determine its effectiveness for you. Continue with that herb if it works or eliminate it if it does not. Experiment with an additional herb if you still need more pain relief, until you find the right combination for you.

- Ginger: Take 100–200 mg three times a day.

- Turmeric: Take 100–300 mg three times a day with meals of a formula that contains 95 percent curcumin.

- Boswellin: Use an extract that contains between 37.5 and 65 percent boswellic acids, and take 200–400 mg three times a day.

- Feverfew: For migraines, use an extract that contains 0.2 percent parthenolids, and take 100–250 mg one to three times a day or eat one to three fresh leaves one to three times daily.

- Holy basil: Brew as a tea or take as dried-leaf capsules. Take one to two grams daily, or follow the directions on the container.

CHAPTER 6

HOMEOPATHIC REMEDIES

Robin, a forty-four-year-old health spa manager, had always been athletic. She loved archery, soccer, squash, volleyball, softball, and tennis. Then she developed chronic knee pain and sciatica—pain so severe that sports were out of the question. She had trouble sleeping and walking down stairs. After an MRI revealed severe osteoarthritis of her knees, her doctor told her that he believed she would never be able to play sports again.

Cut off from the activities that had once given her so much joy, she found herself gaining weight and becoming depressed. It didn't help that she required twelve to fifteen NSAID tablets a day to control her pain, or that she had begun to experience heart palpitations from these excessive doses of pain reliever.

Then a coworker recommended a homeopathic-combination remedy to Robin, telling her that this remedy had worked wonders for her own fibromyalgia pain. Doubtful that such a remedy could really work, but desperate for relief, Robin tried the remedy. She quickly noticed big differences in her level of pain, and within a week was sleeping better. Her mood improved dramatically, and she was able to go back to playing some tennis. She had to keep using the remedy every day, but as long as she did so, her pain was completely gone. Now, she's a firm believer in the power of homeopathy—an area of natural medicine that, to put it mildly, inspires skepticism in many people. On page 78, you will learn what homeopathic ingredients she used.

I have found that when used consistently and appropriately, properly chosen homeopathic remedies can give short-term pain relief, enabling you to keep up with your life until dietary changes and supplements begin to take effect. A number of people with chronic pain have some improvement with natural remedies, but not *complete* relief; if this describes you, homeopathy might be your best bet for addressing day-to-day pain over the long haul as well. In combination with other natural remedies, homeopathy may enable you to achieve complete pain control.

Homeopathics are generally recognized as safe and nontoxic. Such claims of nontoxicity are, of course, not the case for traditional pharmaceutical medicines. Skepticism abounds when it comes to this healing art, but there's no denying that homeopathy has been helpful for many people—even those who didn't believe that it would work for them . . . myself included.

History of Homeopathy

Homeopathy is an art and science developed more than one hundred years ago by a physician named Samuel Hahnemann. Once established, homeopathy became a medical practice used commonly by doctors throughout the United States and Europe until the advent of modern, mainstream pharmaceutical medicine in the first half of the twentieth century. Even though homeopathy is not as popular as it once was in the United States, its popularity has not waned in Europe.

Homeopathy
Homeopathy uses extremely small concentrations of active substances derived from plants, animals, or minerals to counteract symptoms of illness.

Rather than trying to squash disease symptoms by turning off specific biochemical processes in the body, homeopathy relies on the theory of "like cures like." This theory suggests that by introducing exceedingly small concentrations of substances that *cause* specific symptoms in the body, we elicit an opposing response, and the body uses its own resources to relieve those symptoms.

Remember, this is theory, and no one really knows exactly how it works.

Thousands of homeopathic remedies exist, and each one was developed through a scientific homeopathy process known as *proving*. In a proving, healthy subjects are given various homeopathically prepared substances, and their responses are carefully documented. The theory: Whatever symptoms the substances cause in healthy people are the same symptoms that the remedy can be used to relieve in unhealthy people.

While extensive research has not yet been done on homeopathic treatments, there have been some successful studies that support what many people have discovered about the benefits of homeopathy. For example, the company Zicam has recently developed a scientifically tested homeopathic formulation that has become very popular because it decreases the severity and length of time for a cold. Research shows that this remedy can decrease the duration of cold symptoms by up to 75 percent if started within the first twenty-four hours of a cold's onset. A more recent study found that Zicam even helps decrease cold duration if started within forty-eight hours of cold onset. The research shows that there's more to it than the placebo effect.

Homeopathic remedies are considered safe and nontoxic. They are not associated with side effects. While many of the ingredients used homeopathically are toxic before dilution, when diluted down to infinitesimally small amounts of the active ingredients, they become harmless—and healing. For example: A common homeopathic ingredient used for pain control is *Rhus toxicondendron*, which comes from the poison ivy plant. In these small amounts, the remedy never causes poison ivy; instead, it reduces pain in the joints and muscles and has other healing activity as well.

Whether your joint or muscle pain or stiffness is caused by osteoarthritis or swinging your tennis racket too hard; whether it is in your neck or your left big toe—homeopathic remedies for pain can help. Homeopathy is not meant to replace other dietary changes, pain-controlling supplements, or nutrients that promote joint health, just as traditional pharmaceutical pain medications do not. It can, however, relieve pain partly or completely, faster than these other natural methods. The ten homeopathic ingredients discussed in this chapter—*Rhus toxicondendron, Bryonia alba, Ledum palustre,* sulfur, arnica, *Ruta graveolens, Aurum metallicum, Calcarea phosphorica, Apis mellifica, Rhododendron chrysanthum*— are the ones that I have found to be most effective for treating joint and muscle pain, and they can be effective for stiffness and inflammation as well. Combinations of homeopathic ingredients, when carefully chosen, can be very effective. I initially developed this specific combination of these for my own use, but I have also used them in this combination successfully for many patients.

Homeopathy is safe and, when compared to other natural approaches, is fast—and that's what people in pain need so they can get on with their lives and make long-term changes that will help keep pain away for good. It isn't a cure. It's a treatment that can be used without risk, but it's just that— a *treatment* for pain. Healing the underlying problems that are causing that pain will more than likely require nutritional approaches (like those I've recommended in previous chapters) and an intelligently designed exercise program. (See my website, www. DrFranksPainRelief.com, for suggestions about exercise to stop chronic pain, including headaches, or consult with a physical therapist.)

Homeopathic remedies will probably need to be used daily if you are a person with chronic pain, but this is far better than taking traditional pharmaceuticals daily. You still need to use diet and nutritional supplementation as described in this book to help make your joint tissue healthy.

The Homeopathy Controversy

The concept of homeopathy may sound far-fetched to some, and it seemed so to me when I began my own research into the treatments. There are a lot of voices out there that say that homeopathy isn't real science, that it's a hoax, that it's nothing but a placebo effect. I too was a cynic until I put together a unique combination of homeopathic ingredients that worked for me and for my patients to stop joint and muscle pain. Many patients and doctors alike have positive experiences with homeopathy. In fact, a lot of respected physicians who use homeopathy to treat their patients say that although we don't really know exactly how it works, homeopathy does work.

Most evidence of homeopathy's effectiveness is based on personal experience although mainstream medicine tends to dismiss personal experience as supportive evidence in favor of a treatment—after all, it's not the gold standard of traditional medical research, the double-blind, placebo-controlled trial. But in the grand scale of history, medicines have been developed in this way since mankind first began to experiment with medicinal plants. Many of the pharmaceuticals that were first in the *PDR* (*Physicians' Desk Reference*, the key reference book of pharmaceuticals used by physicians), including aspirin, were never subjected to scientific studies. Their merits were established largely through the personal experiences of doctors and patients.

My Own Homeopathy Experience: Doctor Becomes Patient

Several years ago, I developed pain in my neck, upper and lower back, hands, and wrists. Sitting for long hours at my computer was catching up with me, and my existing osteoarthritis was starting to worsen. On top of all this, I developed severe tendonitis in both elbows—a result of what I like to call aggressive gardening, a hobby I have loved since childhood.

Over time, these aches and pains began to increase in intensity, interfering with my daily activities. I knew that NSAIDs weren't safe to overuse, but I needed them to get through the day. I used ibuprofen, aspirin, and naproxen while increasing my intake of certain nutrients and doing helpful stretches. Gradually, I increased my daily use of these drugs just to maintain my normal level of functioning. Eventually, my doctor prescribed a COX-2 inhibitor, and before I knew it, all the medication I was taking caused a bleeding gastric ulcer, and I landed as a patient in my local hospital.

My doctor told me to stop taking NSAIDs and put me on medication to heal my ulcer. I knew I had to find an alternative method for treating my pain. My research led me to homeopathy. After all, this was a hundred-year-old science, and these remedies were well known to be safe and nontoxic. I developed a treatment program for myself that targeted the many kinds of joint and muscle pain I was experiencing.

Even I was skeptical when I began homeopathic treatments. I soon discovered that a unique combination of ten specific homeopathic ingredients worked effectively on my joint and muscle pain, inflammation, and stiffness. Eventually, I used these on many patients and had other doctors do so as well. As expected, based on the homeopathic re - search, this combination of ingredients worked on many different types of chronic joint and muscle pain and stiffness including pain caused from all types of arthritis, temperomandibular joint syndrome (TMJ), tendonitis, fibromyalgia syndrome (FMS), old injuries (fractures and sprains), and other disorders.

The controversy over homeopathy will probably rage for a long time. Science may take centuries more to grasp the biological mechanisms behind its effects—and it may never do so. If you are interested in homeopathy, the best way to decide whether it works for you is to try it for yourself.

Rhus Toxicondendron

Rhus Toxicondendron (*Rhus tox*) is probably the most-recommended homeopathic remedy for pain. As mentioned earlier, it is made from poison ivy. It's useful for arthritis, lower back pain, stiff joints, sprains, strains, and even the intense pain of shingles. According to the homeopathic literature, *Rhus tox* is also a remedy for poison ivy and poison oak—it's a good one to keep in your home first-aid kit.

Bryonia Alba

This treatment, derived from the white bryony vine—a plant that's in the same family as the cucumber—is recommended for pain related to arthritis, joint pain, headache, abdominal pain, back spasms, bone and body aches, sciatica, heartburn, and feverish illnesses.

Ledum Palustre

Derived from a beautiful, white-flowered plant, *Ledum palustre* is a particularly good treatment for pain related to skin wounds or acne. It is also used by homeopaths to soothe pain from arthritis, strains, sprains, and other injuries.

Sulfur

You'll recall that organic sulfur, or MSM, is a useful supplement for pain; homeopathic sulfur is also used for this symptom. Homeopaths believe that it is also good for pain from abscesses (it helps them come to a head and drain) and sore throat.

Arnica (*Arnica Montana*)

For muscle aches and pains, this is the remedy of choice. Arnica, also known as leopard's bane, can be used topically or internally to soothe pain from overwork, sports injury, or arthritis. Midwives recommend it to women with postpartum pain. If you are scheduled for surgery or are planning a big athletic event, homeopaths advise that you can use arnica beforehand to reduce injury and promote faster healing. Arnica cream, rubbed onto painful areas, is one of the most popular homeopathic products and is recommended particularly for shin splints or sore muscles.

Ruta Graveolens

This treatment is made from a small evergreen shrub. It's reported to be effective for bone, joint, and tendon soreness as well as lower back pain, painful deposits or cysts, carpal tunnel syndrome, and pain from eye strain.

Aurum Metallicum

Prescribed for emotional problems related to pain, *Aurum*—a homeopathic form of the mineral gold—is touted to soothe stress and anxiety and helps lift depressed moods.

Calcarea Phosphorica

This homeopathic form of calcium is the top remedy for healthy bones. According to the homeopathic literature, *Calcarea phosphorica* aids in the absorption of dietary calcium and is a popular remedy for headache, "growing pains," teething pain, and arthritis.

Apis Mellifica

Derived from honeybees, this remedy is reported to sooth pain that involves swelling, edema (accumulation of excess fluid), sunburn or other burns, and other itchy, burning types of pain.

Rhododendron Chrysanthum

Derived from the leaves of the golden-flowered rhododendron plant, this treatment is mainly used as a remedy for arthritis pain.

Self-Treating with Homeopathic Remedies

Homeopathy is as much an art as it is a science. A homeopathic practitioner will do a detailed evaluation of a patient in the physical, psychological, and energetic senses to develop a prescription. Typically, the therapeutic value of a visit to a homeopath has a lot to do with the long conversation between healer and patient about what's needed. Some medical doctors also employ homeopathy in their practices. So, too, do many naturopathic doctors.

Remedies are sold in a variety of potencies. The least diluted are the least potent, and the most diluted—up to one hundred dilutions of one part active ingredient to fifty thousand parts water—are the most potent. It is possible to pick out your own homeopathic remedies at the health-food store. Many of these stores have reference books available to help those who wish to self-prescribe homeopathic remedies. Ask a clerk to help you, or invest in a visit to a homeopathic practitioner.

Combination Remedies

Finding just the right homeopathic ingredient—or combination of ingredients—can involve much trial and error. This exploration can take an enormous amount of time and can be expensive if you purchase individual ingredients and try them one at a time. If they don't work for you, you will also be in the unfortunate position of continuing to suffer from chronic pain.

I have tried to reduce the trial-and-error element for my patients by developing a formula that utilizes all of the ten homeopathic ingredients listed in this chapter. This formula has worked very effectively for hundreds of patients with chronic joint and muscle pain and stiffness. The person described in the opening of this chapter used this combination. Some of those patients were also physicians who have then turned around and recommended this combination of homeopathic remedies to their own patients.

Walter, one physician-patient of mine, is in his early seventies. His back, knees, hands, and wrists were getting creaky, and he knew from experience that he was highly sensitive to medications; even buffered aspirin caused side effects so intolerable that he would rather just deal with the joint pain. He recognized that his pain from osteoarthritis was like so many others his age. He characterized his daily pain as moderate to severe, and, as it got progressively worse, it prevented him from enjoying bicycling, swimming, and tennis. Once he started using the combination remedy I recommended, he got the discomfort down to a minimal level. In fact, all of his pains completely disappeared except some minimal pain that occurs at the base of his thumb when he exercises.

Dr. Rick Ajootian is a fibromyalgia specialist in central California. He uses many alternative approaches for his fibromyalgia patients who suffer severe joint and muscle aches and pains daily, and who often don't respond to conventional techniques. He initially tried my recommended homeopathic combination on three patients who were among his most difficult to treat. They all went from experiencing severe pain to reporting mild pain in less than a month, and he is now frequently recommending this combination to his patients.

If you are interested in learning about the homeopathic combination for pain that I discussed in this chapter, visit www.DrFranksPainRelief.com or call 1-800-921-5576. This is a much less expensive way of purchasing this combination than buying each individual ingredient separately.

Dr. Frank's Natural Pain Prescription: Homeopathic Remedies

- Homeopathy is a one-hundred-year-old healing art developed by physician Samuel Hahnemann and is used extensively around the world.

- Do not take homeopathics in place of supplements and dietary modifications. While you can do this, it is better to take them in addition to pain treatment with supplements and diet, both of which benefit the health of the joint tissues.

- Homeopathic remedies can relieve pain and can control it if used consistently.

- The top ten homeopathics for joint and muscle pain relief according to Dr. Frank are *Rhus tox, Bryonia alba, Ledum palustre,* sulfur, arnica, *Ruta graveolens, Aurum metallicum, Calcarea phosphorica, Apis mellifica,* and *Rhododendron chrysanthum.*

CONCLUSION

I hope that what has been laid out in these pages is helpful to you or to your loved one. It's the cream of the current crop of knowledge of how to treat pain by natural means. Let's take a look at the big picture so that you can apply this knowledge to your own health-care journey.

Pain is a messenger that seeks to let you know when something is injured or out of balance in your body. The mainstream methods used to treat it—NSAIDs, COX-2 inhibitors, acetaminophen, corticosteroids, and other drugs—may be necessary and helpful in the short-term and might work faster than natural remedies, but they threaten overall health in the long-term.

Natural pain relievers have track records of safety and effectiveness that stretch back for decades, even millennia. And remember that with the natural approach to pain relief, all roads lead to Rome. Using the natural approach to relieve pain with diet modification and supplements not only reduces pain, but also drastically improves your overall health. Many natural pain remedies used to stop pain also improve cardiovascular health and reduce the risks of cancer and Alzheimer's disease—partly due, in all likelihood, to their anti-inflammatory and antioxidant actions.

A diet rich in omega-3 fats and low in pro-inflammatory omega-6 and hydrogenated fats is the first step and, according to my research, the most powerful dietary way toward reducing inflammation and pain. Eating plenty of vegetables and fruit and avoiding sugars and most grains, and eating foods that are low on the glycemic index, is the second step. Once this anti-inflammatory diet is established, you have set the groundwork for the rest of your program.

A high-potency multivitamin and a few extra nutrients for antioxidant protection will cover any bases your diet misses, ensuring that you are as well nourished as possible. Then, when you use herbal medicines, MSM, glucosamine, chondroitin, ASU, or other nutrients discussed in this book, your body will be ready to use these additional nutrients and herbs to your best advantage.

Turn to homeopathic pain relief when you want to feel better faster than you might by using diet and supplements alone. But don't stop working on finding the best possible long-term plan using diet and supplements to get rid of pain. Your overall health will be better for it.

Don't overlook other aspects of overall health—exercise, weight loss, stress reduction, posture, and biomechanics—in the overall scheme of your pain-relief plan. If you want more information on these topics, visit my web site at www.DrFranksPainRelief.com to investigate them further.

SELECTED REFERENCES

Anon. "Are Ginger and Willow Bark Extracts Viable Alternatives to Treat Osteoarthritis?" *Journal of the American Botanical Council* 55. (2002): 20–24.

Anon. "Fish Oil." Bandolier. http://www.ebandolier.com (April 2005).

Fortin, P.R., et al. "Validation of a meta-analysis: the effects of fish oil in rheumatoid arthritis." *J Clinical Epidemiology* 48. (1995): 1379–1390.

Gescher, A. "Polyphenolic phytochemicals versus nonsteroidal anti-inflammatory drugs: which are better cancer chemopreventive agents?" *Journal of Chemotherapy* 16 Suppl 4. (November 2004): 3–6.

Huemer, R.P., M.D. "Arthritis After Vioxx: The Media's Focus on Prescription Pain Killers Ignores Natural Remedies for Preventing and Treating Arthritis." *LifeExtension Magazine*, February 2005.

Kelm, M.A., et al. "Antioxidant and cyclooxygenase inhibitory phenolic compounds from *Ocimum sanctum linn.*" *Phytomedicine* 1. (March 2000): 7–13.

LaValle, James. *COX-2 Connection: Natural Breakthrough Treatments for Arthritis, Alzheimer's, and Cancer.* Rochester, Vermont: Healing Arts Press, 2001.

Maimes, Steven. "Maimes Report on Holy Basil." Holy Basil—Tulsi. http://www.holy-basil.com Accessed July, 2005.

Majeed, M., et al. *Curcuminoids: Antioxidant Phytonutrients.* Piscataway, NJ: NutriScience Publishers, Inc., 1995.

Majeed, M., et al. *Boswellin: The Anti-Inflammatory Phytonutrient.* Piscataway, NJ: Nutriscience Publishers, Inc., 1996.

Mills, Simon and Bone, Kerry. *Essential Guide to Herbal Safety.* London, England: Elsevier Churchill Livingstone: 2005.

Narayan, S. "Curcumin, a multi-functional chemopreventive agent, blocks growth of colon cancer cells by targeting beta-catenin-mediated transactivation and cell-cell adhesion pathways." *Journal of Molecular Histology* 35(3). (March 2004): 301–307.

Sodhi, V. "Inflammatory conditions and Ayurvedic medicine." *Townsend Letter for Doctors and Patients*, February 1, 2005. http://www.findarticles.com/p/articles/mi_m0ISW/is_259–260/ai_n10299324/print.

Srivastava, K.C., Mustafa, T. "Ginger (*Zingiber officinale*) in rheumatism and musculoskeletal disorders." *Medical Hypotheses* 39(4). (December 1992): 342–348.

Teitelbaum, J. "Best of natural herbal/nutritional pain therapies: highly effective treatments for pain and fatigue." *Townsend Letter for Doctors and Patients*, February 1, 2005, http://www.findarticles.com/p/articles/mi_m0ISW/is_259–260/ai_n10299323.

Vogler, B.K., Pittler, M.H., Ernst, E. "Feverfew as a preventative treatment for migraine: a systematic review." *Cephalalgia* 18(10). (December 1998): 704–708.

Wallace, J.M. "Nutritional and botanical modulation of the inflammatory cascade—eicosanoids, cyclooxygenases, and lipoxygenases—as an adjunct in cancer therapy." *Integrated Cancer Therapeutics* 1(1). (March 2002): 7–37.

Yang, F., et al. "Curcumin inhibits formation of amyloid beta oligomers and fibrils, binds plaques, and reduces amyloid in vivo." *Journal of Biological Chemistry* 280(7). (February 2005): 5892–5901.

OTHER BOOKS
AND RESOURCES

Books

The Inflammation Syndrome: The Complete Nutritional Program to Prevent and Reverse Heart Disease, Arthritis, Diabetes, Allergies, and Asthma (Wiley, 2003) by Jack Challem. A wonderful overview of inflammation's role in disease and how to control it naturally. Dr. Frank's favorite source for guidance in shopping, meals and eating at restaurants.

The Omega Diet: The Lifesaving Nutritional Program Based on the Diet of the Island of Crete (Collins/Harper Perennial) by Artemis P. Simopoulos and Jo Robinson. A great primer on omega-3 fats.

Nourishing Traditions: The Cookbook that Challenges Politically Correct Nutrition and the Diet Dictocrats by Sally Fallon (NewTrends Publishing, 1999). More on the Stone Age approach; well written with plenty of recipes.

The Anti-Inflammation Zone: Reversing the Silent Epidemic That's Destroying Our Health by Barry Sears (ReganBooks, 2005). The eicosanoid master contributes his ten cents' worth on the inflammation issue.

The Arthritis Foundation's Guide to Pain Management: Natural and Medical Therapies by Sarah Bernstein (Arthritis Foundation, 2003).

The Arthritis Foundation's Guide to Living Well With Rheumatoid Arthritis by Gretchen Henkel (Arthritis Foundation, 2003).

Fibromyalgia and Chronic Myofascial Pain: A Survival Manual (2nd Edition) by Mary Ellen Copeland (New Harbinger Publications, 2001).

The Headache Prevention Cookbook: Eating Right to Prevent Migraine and Other Headaches (Houghton Mifflin, 2000) by David R. Marks and Laura Marks.

Managing Pain Before It Manages You (The Guilford Press, 2001) by Margaret A. Caudill, M.D., Ph.D. A nice overview of using your mind to help relieve pain in your body.

Healing Back Pain: The Mind-Body Connection (Warner Books, 1991) and *The MindBody Prescription: Healing the Body, Healing the Pain* (Warner Books, 1999), both by John E. Sarno, M.D. Tells us how tension and pain cooperate to keep us hurting and how to break the cycle.

Encyclopedia of Natural Medicine (Three Rivers Press, 1997) by Michael Murray, N.D., and Joseph Pizzorno, N.D., and its companion book, *Encyclopedia of Nutritional Supplements* (Three Rivers Press, 1996) by Michael Murray, N.D. A great overall resource on natural medicines, particularly nutrient supplementation.

The Miracle of MSM: The Natural Solution for Pain (Berkeley Trade, 1999) by Stanley W. Jacob, M.D., Ronald M. Lawrence, M.D., Ph.D., and Martin Zucker. *The* book on MSM by the man who has most intensively researched its use as a pain medicine.

The Arthritis Cure: The Medical Miracle That Can Halt, Reverse, and May Even Cure Osteoarthritis (St. Martin's Griffin, 2004) by Jason Theosodakis, M.D., M.S., MPH, FACPM, and Sheila Buff. Lots of information on supplements for osteoarthritis.

The Green Pharmacy: The Ultimate Compendium of Natural Remedies from the World's Foremost Authority on Healing Herbs (St. Martin's Paperbacks, 1998) by James A. Duke. A witty and warm reference book for herb novices and experts alike.

The Complete Homeopathy Handbook: Safe and Effective Ways to Treat Fevers, Coughs, Colds and Sore Throats, Childhood Ailments, Food Poisoning, Flu, and a Wide Range of Everyday Complaints (St. Martin's Griffin, 1991) by Miranda Castro. A good resource for your health library.

Websites

The Dietary Supplement Information Bureau runs a helpful site at www.supplementinfo.org.

Herbs by Name, a web site run by the University of Maryland, can be found at umm.edu/altmed/ConsLookups/Herbs.html.

Dr. Frank's Pain Relief website sells his homeopathic pain relief oral spray and provides additional information about natural approaches to stop pain including information about headache control and exercises to stop chronic pain. Go to www.DrFranksPainRelief.com or call 1-800-220-7687.

Nutrition Online is a website of Dr. Frank's that provides information on Advanced Physicians' Products and natural healing, including a large variety of nutritional supplements. Go to www.nutritiononline.com or call (800) 220-7687.

The National Center for Homeopathy has information on homeopathy on their site at www.homeopathic.org.

Magazines

Let's Live Magazine
Consumer magazine with emphasis on the health benefits of vitamins, minerals, and herbs.
Customer service:
1-800-676-4333
P.O. Box 74908
Los Angeles, CA 90004
Subscriptions: 12 issues per year, $19.95 in the U.S.; $31.95 outside the U.S.

Physical Magazine
Magazine oriented to body builders and other serious athletes.
Customer service:
1-800-676-4333
P.O. Box 74908
Los Angeles, CA 90004
Subscriptions: 12 issues per year, $19.95 in the U.S.; $31.95 outside the U.S.

The Nutrition Reporter™ newsletter

Monthly newsletter that summarizes recent medical research on vitamins, minerals, and herbs. (A favorite of Dr. Frank's.)

Customer service:

P.O. Box 30246

Tucson, AZ 85751-0246

e-mail: jack@thenutritionreporter.com

www.nutritionreporter.com

Subscriptions: $26 per year (12 issues) in the U.S.; $32 U.S. or $48 CNC for Canada; $38 for other countries

INDEX

diet and, 15–27
herbs for, 59–69
symptoms, 17
Inositol, 33
Insulin, 21, 23
resistance, 23
Interleukin-12, 61
Iodine, 33
Irritable bowel syndrome
(IBS), 25

*Journal of the American
Medical Association*, 29
Junk food, 18, 19

LA, 20
Lancet, The, 52
Leaky gut syndrome, 11
Ledum Palustre, 76
Leukotrienes, 64
Licorice, 68
Linoleic acid. *See* LA.
Lipoic acid. *See* Alpha lipoic
acid.
Lupus, 35
Lutein, 48
Lycopene, 48

Macadamia nut oil, 26, 27
Magnesium, 33
Manganese, 33
Medical College of Virginia,
52
Mega-Zyme, 33
Menstrual pain, 4, 9, 14, 36, 63
Metabolic syndrome. *See*
Syndrome X.
Methylsulfonylmethane
(MSM), 43–44, 49, 56, 76,
82
Migraine, 4, 8–9, 14, 42, 63,
66
Milk products. *See* Dairy
products.
Molybdenum, 33
Morphine, 2, 13
MSM. *See*
Methylsulfonylmethane
(MSM).
Musculoskeletal syndrome.
See Fibromyalgia.

N-acetylcysteine (NAC), 48
Natural medicine, 2–3

*New Glucose Revolution
Guide to Glycemic Index*,
24
Niacin. *See* Vitamin B$_3$.
NSAIDs, 5–6, 10–11, 13, 14,
17–18, 36, 50, 53, 55,
56–57, 59–60, 63, 67, 68,
70, 75, 81
heart failure and, 13
Nutrient chart, 48–49
Nutrition. *See* Diet.
Nutritional supplements. *See*
Supplements.
Nuts, 25–26

Oils, hydrogenated, 18, 19, 22
Olive oil, 26, 27
Omega-3 fatty acids, 7, 18,
19–23, 26, 27, 34, 47, 81
Omega-6 fatty acids, 19–22,
26, 27, 34, 39, 42, 47, 81
Omega-9 fatty acids, 26
Omega Rx, 39
Opiates, 13
Organic sulfur. *See* Methyl-
sulfonylmethane (MSM).
Osteoarthritis, 4, 5, 14, 35, 42,
50–53, 63, 70, 72, 74, 79
Osteoporosis, 36
Overuse injuries, 4

Pain, 1–3, 4–14, 15–27, 28–49,
50–57, 59–69, 70–80, 81–82
antioxidants and, 44–47
diet and, 15–27
herbs for, 58–69
homeopathic remedies,
70–80
inflammation and, 15–27
mainstream treatments,
4–14
supplemental nutrients
and, 28–49
types that do not respond
to natural therapies, 4
types that respond to
natural therapies, 4
vitamins and, 28–49
Pain Net, Inc., 1
Pancreas, 23
Parthenolides, 66
Pathogens, 16
*Physicians' Desk Reference
(PDR)*, 74

Printed in the USA
CPSIA information can be obtained
at www.ICGtesting.com
JSHW012008140824
68134JS00004B/59